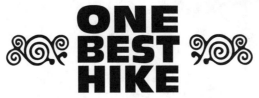

ONE BEST HIKE

MOUNT RAINIER'S WONDERLAND TRAIL

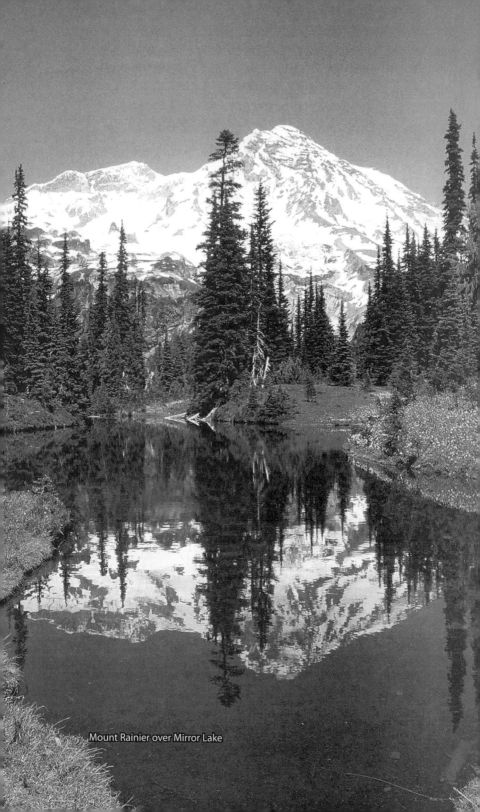
Mount Rainier over Mirror Lake

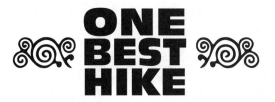

ONE BEST HIKE

MOUNT RAINIER'S WONDERLAND TRAIL

Everything you need to know to successfully hike all the way around this great mountain

Douglas Lorain

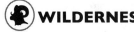 **WILDERNESS PRESS** . . . *on the trail since 1967*

One Best Hike: Mount Rainier's Wonderland Trail

1st EDITION

Copyright © 2012 by Douglas Lorain
All cover and interior photos, unless otherwise noted, by Douglas Lorain
Cover design: Larry B. Van Dyke and Scott McGrew
Book design and layout: Andreas Schueller and Annie Long
Cartography: Douglas Lorain
Editor: Amber Kaye Henderson

Library of Congress Cataloging-in-Publication Data

Lorain, Douglas, 1962-
 One best hike : Mount Rainier's Wonderland Trail / by Douglas Lorain.
-- 1st ed.
   p. cm.
 Includes index.
 ISBN 978-0-89997-655-6 -- ISBN 0-89997-655-7
 1. Hiking--Washington (State)--Wonderland Trail--Guidebooks. 2.
Hiking--Washington (State)--Mount Rainier National Park--Guidebooks.
3. Wonderland Trail (Wash.)--Guidebooks. 4. Mount Rainier National
Park (Wash.)--Guidebooks. I. Title.
 GV199.42.W22W654 2012
 796.5109797--dc23
                          2012018030

Manufactured in the United States of America

Published by: **Wilderness Press**
                 c/o Keen Communications
                 PO Box 43673
                 Birmingham, AL 35243
                 (800) 443-7227
                 info@wildernesspress.com
                 www.wildernesspress.com

Visit our website for a complete listing of our books and for ordering information.

Distributed by Publishers Group West

SAFETY NOTICE: Although Wilderness Press and the author have made every attempt to ensure that the information in this book is accurate at press time, they are not responsible for any loss, damage, injury, or inconvenience that may occur to anyone while using this book. Readers are advised to recheck phone numbers, prices, addresses, and other material. You are responsible for your own safety and health while in the wilderness. The fact that a trail is described in this book does not mean that it will be safe for you. The potential for falls, heat exhaustion, dehydration, hyperventilation, or other problems are possible (though not likely). Be aware that trail conditions can change from day to day. Always check local conditions and the weather, and know your own limitations.

Acknowledgments

The help of many people made this book possible. Special thanks go to the following persons:

National Park Service personnel who provided information, read drafts, or otherwise shared their considerable expertise: Scott Beason, Dan Camiccia, Craig Cope, Geoff Walker, and James Ziolkowski.

The people at Wilderness Press/Keen Communications who continue to enthusiastically publish my books and do such a stellar job of turning my initial disjointed writing and mapping efforts into something usable and attractive for you, the reader. On this book, particular thanks go to Amber Kaye Henderson, Scott McGrew, and Molly Merkle.

Most of all, as always, I thank my wife, Becky Lovejoy, who stoically endured much time alone taking care of the dog and house while her husband traipsed off into the wilds of Mount Rainier. Her love and encouragement are invaluable to this book and to my life.

While the contributions and assistance of the persons listed above were significant, all of the text, maps, and photos herein are my own work and sole responsibility. Any and all omissions, errors, and just plain stupid mistakes are strictly mine.

Douglas Lorain

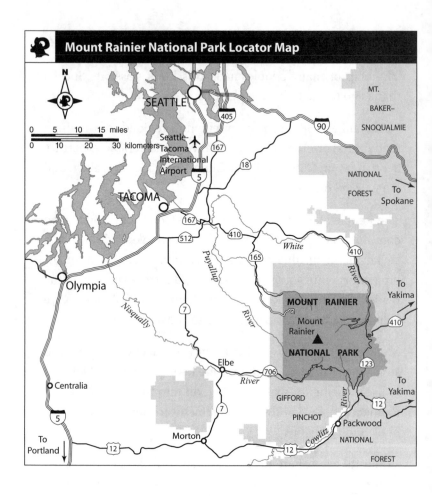

Mount Rainier National Park Locator Map

Contents

List of Maps

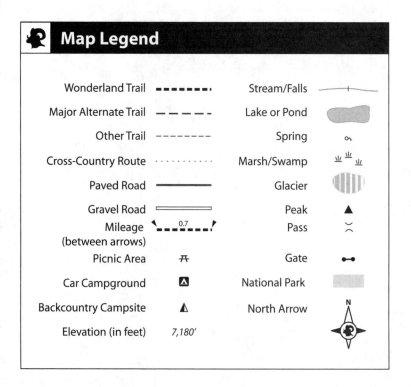

Map Legend			
Wonderland Trail		Stream/Falls	
Major Alternate Trail		Lake or Pond	
Other Trail		Spring	
Cross-Country Route		Marsh/Swamp	
Paved Road		Glacier	
Gravel Road		Peak	▲
Mileage (between arrows)	0.7	Pass	
Picnic Area	🏕	Gate	
Car Campground		National Park	
Backcountry Campsite	▲	North Arrow	
Elevation (in feet)	7,180'		

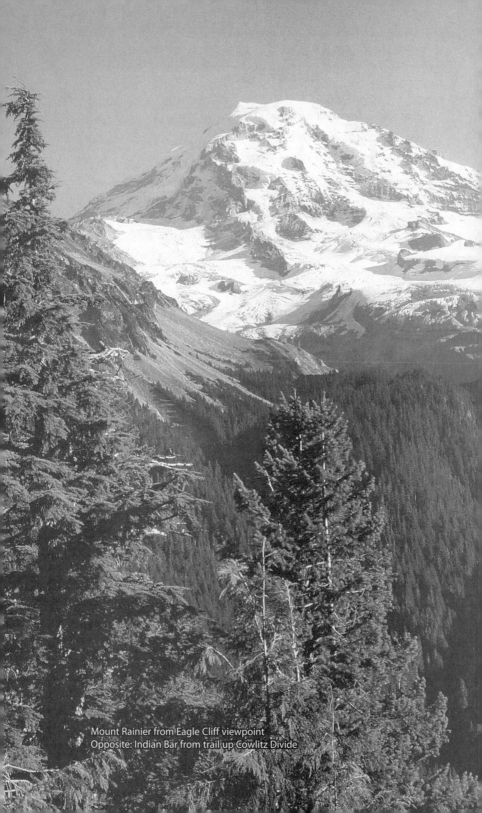

Mount Rainier from Eagle Cliff viewpoint
Opposite: Indian Bar from trail up Cowlitz Divide

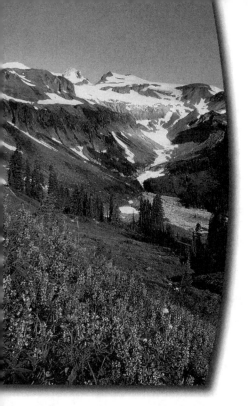

Introduction

"Mt. Rainier, or Tahoma (the Indian name), is the noblest of the volcanic cones extending from Lassen Butte and Mt. Shasta along the Cascade Range to Mt. Baker. . . . Rainier . . . surpasses them all in massive icy grandeur—the most majestic solitary mountain I had ever yet beheld."

—John Muir,
Travels in Alaska, 1915

Mount Rainier and the Wonderland Trail

A s any Seattle area resident looking up and admiring "their" mountain can attest, John Muir, as usual, had it right. Mount Rainier is truly a majestic sight that dominates its surroundings like no other peak in the lower 48 United States. Given the mountain's size and prominence, it is not surprising that this geographic wonder is defined by superlatives. It is the tallest mountain in the state of Washington, and, for that matter, in the entire Cascade Range, making it the undisputed king of the Pacific Northwest. It supports (by far) the largest glacier system of any mountain in the United States, outside of Alaska, and proudly displays its permanent mantle of white to awed viewers who are as far as 100 miles away in every direction (at least on days when clouds don't block the view). It is protected in what was only our nation's fifth, and what is still one of its best, national parks, established all the way back in 1899. It is the largest volcanic mountain in the lower 48 United States and one of the largest in the world. It supports thriving populations of some of the continent's most impressive wildlife and grandest trees, as well as some of the most abundant displays of wildflowers of any area in the country. And, admittedly more of an opinion than a quantifiable fact, it is simply one of the most beautiful and awe-inspiring peaks you will find anywhere.

But, for all that, this book is not about the mountain itself. Instead, this book highlights what is, in the opinion of thousands of amazed pedestrians over the years, the best way to see, feel, and appreciate this grand mountain: hiking all the way around it.

Like the mountain it encircles, the Wonderland Trail is defined by superlatives. With a length of 92.2 miles (or thereabouts, depending on which measurement you believe) and, perhaps more significant, with nearly *4 vertical miles of uphill* along the way, this is one of the longest and toughest trails in the entire national park system. The trail passes through every life zone in the park, so hikers enjoy everything from cathedral stands of low-elevation old-growth rain forest to starkly beautiful above-timberline landscapes of rocks and glaciers. In between are numerous waterfalls, some of the grandest mountain wildflower displays in the world, plenty of wildlife, dozens of small lakes, idyllic mountain meadows, rushing glacial torrents spanned by frightening swinging bridges, meandering clear brooks crossed by quaint logs, and countless opportunities for side trips to little-known glories high on the slopes of the mountain. It is hardly surprising, then, that virtually every list of the greatest hikes in North America places the Wonderland Trail near the top.

For any avid backpacker the Wonderland Trail is a hike on his or her life list that should be taken at least once before the body decides that the heavy backpack has to be put away for good. For more than a few locals, the trail is not a one-time thing but an annual adventure, with the ever-changing scenery drawing them back year after year to this mountain pilgrimage. The fact that you are reading this book probably means that you would like to join this cadre of satisfied hikers, adding the Wonderland Trail to your own list of lifetime best hikes. With the help of this book, you are cordially invited to do just that. In addition to being a complete trail guide that fully describes the main trail, several excellent alternate routes, and dozens of the best side trips, this book guides you through the often complex planning and logistics required by this daunting hike. The goal is to make your trip not only more enjoyable but also easier to complete and to ensure that once you take those final steps back to your car at (probably) Longmire, you won't be disappointed.

Mount Rainier's Human History

Today's hikers are far from the first to appreciate the value and wonders of Mount Rainier. Although the archaeological evidence is sketchy, based on studies in other parts of the Cascade Range, human beings have probably been visiting the area now occupied by Mount Rainier National Park for as long as 8,000 years. Most of the park has not been thoroughly surveyed, but several dozen known sites indicate that Native Americans used the area for hunting, tool stone procurement, and the gathering of berries and other foods. In historic times, five Native American tribes used the area: the Nisqually, Puyallup, Muckleshoot, Yakama, and Taidnapam. Some of these people continued to visit the park for hunting and berry collection into the early 20th century. Different tribes undoubtedly had different names for the peak, but the generally accepted name in use at the time that Europeans arrived was Tacoma or Tahoma. The word is believed to be from the Lushootseed

A CONTRARIAN'S VIEW

Partly because the authors can hardly be described as unbiased observers, hiking guidebooks rarely present a dissenting view about the beauty and virtues of the trails described in their pages. Because I feel absolutely confident that any rational person will loudly extol the virtues of the Wonderland Trail once he or she hikes its 92 (or so) spectacular miles, I am going to break with tradition and pass along the thoughts of a person who apparently wasn't so enthralled. The managing editor of a prominent hiking magazine (a man who really should know better) once wrote the following about the Wonderland Trail: "Hike around a mountain, suffering all the ups and downs of its ridges and valleys, slogging through constant wet, not getting more than one or two excellent views a day, and not then also climb the damn thing? That's like getting a Blowpop and only consuming the stick."

Not that I want to pick a fight or anything, but with all due respect to this man, he is a blind idiot who doesn't belong on *any* trail without adult supervision. First of all, he must have lost track while trying to count them on his fingers, but the Wonderland Trail offers *hundreds* of great viewpoints, and they come along *far* more frequently than once or twice a day. Second, while it is certainly true that hiking the Wonderland Trail is a strenuous endeavor that requires plenty of climbing over ridges and dropping into valleys, that is all part of hiking. If this man wants to see great scenery without having to work for it, he should stay home on the couch and watch the National Geographic Channel. Finally, if he wants to climb Mount Rainier *in addition* to hiking the Wonderland Trail, then go right ahead. There are climbing services that do just that, and you can get a permit at any of the wilderness information centers in the park (as of 2012 there is a $43 fee for an annual climbing pass, plus $20 for an advance reservation—strongly advised, because this is very popular). It is an amazing experience, and I encourage every reader of this book to learn basic mountain-climbing skills and take a guided sojourn to the summit. But the two experiences—climbing the peak and hiking around it—have nothing to do with one another. My wife and I recently visited the big island of Hawaii. We swam with green sea turtles, hiked across a recently active volcanic crater, visited a spectacular tropical botanical garden, saw lots of interesting birds, and relaxed on idyllic sandy beaches, but I did not have time to climb to the top of Mauna Loa. Does that omission mean that the rest of our trip was somehow bad or a waste of time? I would strongly suggest that this magazine editor have both his eyesight checked and his attitude adjusted.

language spoken by the Puyallups and meant either "mother of waters," "snowcapped peak," or, somewhat less poetically, "larger than Koma," which was the name for another area volcano, the somewhat smaller Mount Baker.

The first Europeans to see Mount Rainier were members of a British exploring expedition under the command of Captain George Vancouver. They sighted the mountain in May 1792, and their captain named the peak after a friend of his, Rear Admiral Peter Rainier of the British Navy. In 1806 members of the Meriwether Lewis and William Clark expedition became the first known American explorers to see the mountain, though they never got closer than the Columbia River, some 80 miles away.

Many of the names of glaciers, peaks, and other geographic features in the park date back to the early explorers who visited the mountain. In 1833, for example, William Tolmie, the physician at the Hudson's Bay Company's Fort Nisqually, became the first known white man to visit the area now occupied by the park when he hired five native guides and came into what is now the northwest corner of the park in search of medicinal plants. Then in 1857 August Valentine Kautz, an Army lieutenant stationed at Fort Steilacoom, made the first documented attempt to climb the mountain. He and some companions hired a Nisqually as a guide and took six days to travel through the nearly impenetrable lower-elevation forests before they finally reached open terrain and began their attempt on the summit. Two days and much hard work later, Kautz made it the farthest of the group, probably topping out at close to 14,000 feet near the ironically titled Point Success (just a little more than 400 feet from the top), but he did not achieve his goal.

In 1859 James Longmire, an ambitious settler to the Washington Territory from Indiana, established the rugged Packwood Trail, which allowed people to travel from the Puget Sound coastline to the lower reaches of Mount Rainier. Fully 11 years later, three of those visitors, guided by Longmire and a Native American named Sluiskin, set out to reach the top. On August 17, 1870, two of those men, Hazard Stevens and Philemon B. Van Trump (Don't you just love those old names? When was the last time you met anybody with a name like Hazard or Philemon?) became the first people to make it to the summit. In 1883, at the for-his-time relatively advanced age of 63, the ever-enterprising Longmire made his first climb to the top of the mountain and, on his way back from that trip, discovered a meadow with some interesting soda and mineral springs. He built a rough-log hotel there and set about convincing people (with considerable success) that soaking in the spring water was a medicinal cure. The meadow, springs, and development he started still carry Longmire's name and today are the most popular starting point for those doing the Wonderland Trail.

One other historical visitor of note was the great conservationist John Muir. Upon seeing the mountain during a visit to Puget Sound in 1888, the excited Muir decided to alter his original travel plans and climb the alluring peak. He succeeded in reaching the summit, although, expressing the same opinion as countless Wonderland Trail visitors since, Muir decided that the peak was best appreciated and more impressive from below than from the top. His writings, along with the images taken by his companion, photographer Arthur C. Warner, helped to bring broader attention to the mountain and its beauty.

On March 2, 1899, following promotion and preservation efforts that began as early as 1883, President William McKinley signed the law creating Mount Rainier as our nation's fifth national park.

At the time of the park's creation, there were already many miles of trails in the area. Most of these were old Native American paths, miner's routes, and trails to favored hunting and food-gathering sites. In addition, Longmire, after establishing his hotel and health spa, had built several trails in the park's southwest corner. There was not, however, any developed trail all the way around the mountain.

Despite the practical difficulties, the *idea* of walking the entire distance around this towering landmark had great appeal, and it was members of a new organization (what would become the Mountaineers, which started in 1906) who helped to promote the idea with their annual sojourns to the peak. In anticipation of a planned trek by members of the group, several unfinished segments of the around-the-mountain route were hastily completed in the summer of 1914 and early in 1915. So it was in the summer of 1915 that 100 Mountaineers made the first recorded expedition around the peak. It was not until 1921, however, that today's wonderfully evocative name for the trail was used in a National Park Service (NPS) report. For obvious reasons, the language stuck and the Wonderland Trail was born.

Natural History

Any visitor to a grand natural playground and outdoor laboratory such as Mount Rainier National Park will (or at least should) be interested in learning about the plants, animals, and rocks that surround them. Most people enjoy their visit much more when they can put a name to the things they see and better understand how those elements fit together in an intricate ecological balance. For the hiker, there is no better way to appreciate the enormous natural diversity of the region than by hiking the Wonderland Trail, because that pathway visits almost every major ecosystem in the park, from lowland forests to alpine meadows and rock gardens. This section provides an overview of the fascinating natural history of the park. Interested hikers are strongly encouraged to learn more by talking to rangers, visiting park museums, and reading any of several excellent books about the area's wildflowers, trees, shrubs, birds, mammals, glaciers, and volcanic eruptions (see Appendix A, on page 181, for recommended reading).

GEOLOGY

As even a casual glance by the uninitiated quickly indicates, the geologic history of Mount Rainier is dominated by the forces of volcanism and glaciers. Mount Rainier is one of

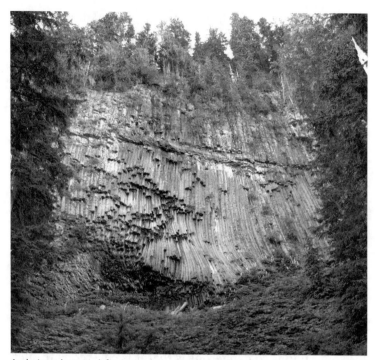

Andesite column rock formation below South Puyallup Camp

the world's most massive stratovolcanoes, built up in a series of lava flows and eruptions over thousands of years. All of the dominant rocks in the park are volcanic in origin, including large amounts of andesite and basalt. Early lava deposits that helped to form the mountain are estimated to be more than 840,000 years old, but the present cone is thought to be a little more than 500,000 years old. Countless eruptions, debris flows, landslides, and lahars (volcanic mudflows) have built up and torn down sections of the peak over the millennia, so its shape and profile have constantly changed over time.

One of the last really large mudflow events was the Osceola Mudflow, which occurred about 5,600 years ago. During this event a large section of the mountain's summit collapsed, removing some 1,600 feet from the top of the peak and sending half a cubic mile of debris down the White River Valley. The unstoppable slurry of mud, debris, and glacial ice flowed downstream and covered most of the present-day city of Tacoma. In the process, the flow undoubtedly killed many Native Americans who were, at that time, living around Puget Sound. Since then, there have been countless smaller mud and debris flows, and these continue to occur today. Debris flows have raced down the canyon of Tahoma Creek, for example, as many as two dozen times since the late 1960s. And in 1963 a massive debris avalanche peeled off the slopes of a side peak called Little Tahoma, rocketed down the Emmons Glacier, and nearly wiped out the White River Campground. Fears about a repeat of the Osceola Mudflow, or any of several possible smaller catastrophes, have placed Mount Rainier at the top of the list of the most dangerous volcanoes in the United States. Part of the reason the mountain is so dangerous is that it is covered with such enormous quantities of ice, which could suddenly melt in an eruption and create massive flooding. Another factor that concerns geologists, as well as local disaster-preparedness officials, is the sheer number of people (hundreds of thousands) who now live in areas that could be devastated by an eruption or even by events such as landslides and mudflows that are not necessarily related to eruptive activity.

Though quiet for now, Mount Rainier is still an active volcano. Continuing geothermal heat keeps areas along the summit rim free of ice and has created both a meltwater lake below the ice and an extensive glacial cave network in the mountain's two summit craters. Reliable eyewitness reports indicate eruptions in 1820, 1846, 1854, 1858, 1879, 1882, and 1894. As of 2012 there is no immediate concern about an eruption, but geologists would not be surprised if the mountain began acting up again.

The second dominant force in shaping the landscape around Mount Rainier is glaciers. These massive, slow-moving rivers of ice gradually carve into, grind up, and carry away huge quantities of rock, leaving behind deep U-shaped valleys, cirque lakes, moraines, and other characteristic features. Today some 25 major glaciers cover approximately 35 square miles of the mountain's surface, so the influence of these icy monsters is ongoing. In the not-so-distant past, much more of the mountain and surrounding area was under ice. During the most recent glacial period, which ended more than 10,000 years ago, glaciers covered virtually every square inch of what is now Mount Rainier National

Mount Rainier and snout of Carbon Glacier

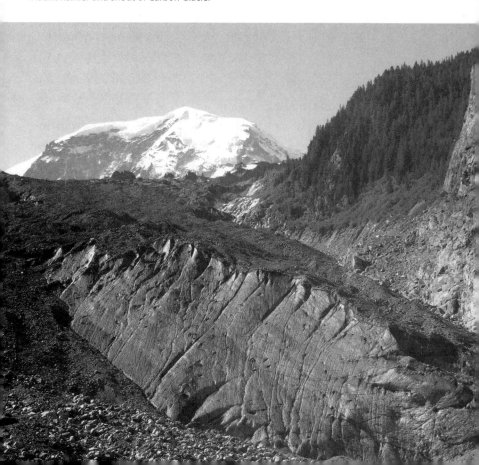

Park. They even extended down from the mountain all the way to the Puget Sound Basin. Then, during the so-called Little Ice Age, between the 14th century and about 1850, the mountain's glaciers advanced again, extending, at times, several miles beyond their current locations. Since then, the glaciers have generally been in an uneven state of retreat, with periodic advances, such as in the late 1970s and early 1980s. Today, most of the mountain's glaciers are thinning and retreating at a relatively rapid rate.

A final important factor in carving the landscape around Mount Rainier is the erosive action of the many creeks and rivers that pour off the mountain. These streams inexorably carry away the sand and debris created by glaciers (for proof, look at the heavily silt-laden creeks and rivers you cross along the trail) and slowly carve deep canyons of their own into the tough volcanic rock.

FLORA

Due to the area's abundant moisture and the park's dramatic and relatively rapid changes in elevation—from just 1,700 feet at the Carbon River to 14,410 feet at the summit (that's almost two-and-a-half times the depth of the Grand Canyon)—the vegetation of Mount Rainier National Park is diverse, lush, and beautiful. Well more than 1,100 species of plants—ranging from fungi and lichens to grasses and sedges, numerous species of ferns, hundreds of different wildflowers, several types of shrubs and small trees, and a number of giant coniferous tree species—live here. Because the Wonderland Trail visits all of the park's vegetation zones, you will have the opportunity during your trip to see virtually all of this incredible diversity of greenery.

About 58% of the park is covered by forest. At the lowest elevations, generally below 2,700 feet, are the giant old

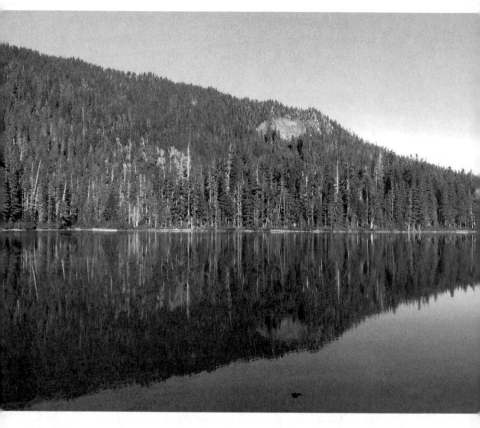

Lake James

specimens of western hemlocks, Douglas firs, and western red cedars. Understory trees in this environment must survive in a land of very little light because the canopy above blocks most of the sunlight from reaching the forest floor. Look in these shady areas for Pacific yews, grand firs, and vine maples. The most abundant ground cover species here include devil's club, thimbleberry, sword and deer ferns, oxalis, and salal. On the few open slopes at these lower elevations, which are kept clear of large trees by frequent avalanches, are dense thickets of alders. Almost 100 species of moss and 200 types of fungi abound in the lush and damp low-elevation environment.

Some of the oldest and largest of the trees in this zone are found along the lower reaches of Ipsut Creek and near the banks of the Carbon River, both in the park's northwest corner and in the Grove of the Patriarchs, just a short side trip off the Eastside alternative to the Wonderland Trail.

As you climb into the midelevation forest zone, which fills the area from 2,700 feet to 4,000–6,000 feet depending on local conditions, you encounter a different mix of conifers. The most notable species here are Pacific silver firs, Alaska yellow cedars, western white pines, and noble firs. The trees here are generally smaller than those at lower elevations, but the forests are usually more diverse in size and age. One of the most delightful understory species in this zone is the huckleberry, which provides a tasty feast in late summer.

Above the forests are the subalpine parklands, which spectacularly host so much of the Wonderland Trail. These make up about 23% of the park's area and include many of the park's most popular road-accessible locations, such as Paradise and Sunrise. Here trees come only in scattered clumps, so you are no longer in forest. Instead the dominant vegetation is grasses, sedges, low-growing shrubs, and amazingly abundant wildflowers. What trees exist are often picturesquely contorted by wind and heavy snowfall and include whitebark pines, mountain hemlocks, subalpine firs, Alaska yellow cedars, and a few Engelmann spruces.

One of the things for which Mount Rainier is justly famous is the abundance and beauty of its wildflowers. In mid- to late summer many visitors are more impressed with the blossoms found carpeting the subalpine parklands than they are with the mountain views. Peak blooming times vary with the elevation and the depth of the previous winter's snowpack, but if seeing lots of wildflowers is part of your reason for hiking the Wonderland Trail, then it's usually best to schedule your hike from very late July to mid-August.

A complete list of the park's wildflowers is beyond the scope of this book (not to mention the expertise of the author), so what follows is only a partial listing of the most abundant species you are likely to encounter. White flowers you should look for include twinflowers, bunchberries, mountain bistorts, Sitka valerians, avalanche lilies, bear grass, western pasqueflowers, pussytoes, yarrows, and, in very moist areas, marsh marigolds. Common yellow and orange wildflowers are glacier lilies, groundsels, fanleaf cinquefoils, buttercups, and orange agoseris (or orange mountain dandelions). Some of the most abundant blue wildflowers are subalpine lupines, larkspurs, bluebells, and, in late summer, gentians. Finally a few of the more abundant red and pink wildflowers are paintbrushes, shooting stars, mountain spireas, pink heather,

Western pasqueflowers

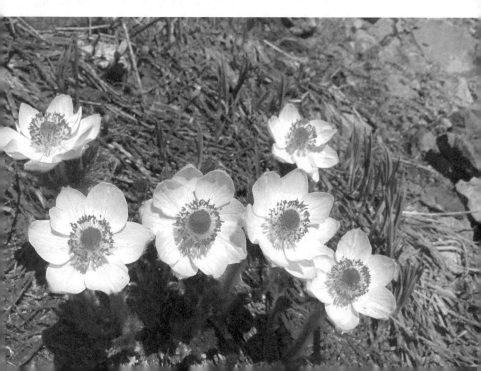

fireweeds, cliff penstemons, and columbines. Anyone who is interested in wildflowers should carry an identification guide. With one of these in hand you could easily spend several happy hours in almost any meadow identifying, photographing, smelling, and generally enjoying the vast array of blossoms that carpet these bits of mountain paradise. Keep in mind, however, that these high meadows have very short growing seasons and are extremely fragile. Always remain on established trails to avoid trampling the delicate flowers.

Above the subalpine parklands is the alpine zone, which is dominated by rocks, ice, and snowfields. Here the plants must cope with extreme conditions and are often very small and hard to see. Tiny rock gardens brighten these areas, and discovering these little patches of color is a real joy. Aster, heather, partridgefoot, moss campion, phlox, and Cusick's speedwell are among the more commonly encountered wildflowers. Other flora include lichens (a favorite food of mountain goats), grasses, and various sedges. Despite the harsh conditions, the plant communities here are among the oldest in the park. Some heather communities, for example, are believed to have persisted in these alpine environments for as long as 10,000 years.

FAUNA

As is true throughout the world, by far the most abundant group of animals in Mount Rainier National Park is the invertebrates—insects, worms, spiders, and the like. Apart from admiring a few colorful butterflies or cursing the blasted mosquitoes, however, most people show little interest in the vast range of little critters. Still, they are vitally important to the health of the park's ecosystems and can be quite fascinating. They range from such unusual animals as ice worms, which live in the mountain's glacial ice, to an array of beetles that prowl the forest floor. Take some time during your hike to examine these miniature beings and appreciate their beauty and importance. (OK, feel free to swat a mosquito or two, but the rest of the group is generally harmless and worth your respect.)

Reptiles, which generally prefer warmer and drier habitats than what predominates at Mount Rainier, are fairly rare. Some garter snakes and rubber boas, as well as a few northern alligator lizards, live in the park, but that pretty much completes the list. Amphibians, on the other hand, are abundant. In fact, in many of the park's forest habitats, the biomass (total weight) of amphibians is thought to exceed that of all other vertebrate groups combined. Observant hikers stand a good chance of spotting many species of frogs and salamanders, including western toads, tailed frogs, Cascades frogs, long-toed and Pacific giant salamanders, and rough-skinned newts. One concern when it comes to amphibians is the introduction of fish into lakes that evolved without them. In particular, predation by introduced trout is thought to be responsible for the elimination of many salamander species from several of the park's lakes.

Birds are perhaps the most conspicuous group of animals noticed by park visitors. Several dozen species regularly use the park either as permanent residents or as transients that migrate through the area or that arrive in the spring to nest through the summer months. Almost every hiker is sure to see such abundant and conspicuous species as Steller's jays, common ravens, Clark's nutcrackers, and dark-eyed juncos. With more careful observation you will notice that the different species typically stay in particular habitats found in the park's distinct life zones. With this knowledge it becomes easier to know what to look for in each environment and to identify the types of feathered friends you encounter. In the park's low-elevation forests, for example, you should keep an eye out for red-breasted nuthatches, brown creepers, varied thrushes, winter wrens, hairy woodpeckers, chestnut-backed chickadees, and olive-sided flycatchers. Very lucky and observant visitors may see the threatened northern spotted owl, which makes its home in these dense forests. Birds that are characteristic of the midelevation forests include Wilson's and yellow-rumped warblers, golden-crowned kinglets, hermit thrushes, pine siskins, blue grouses, mountain chickadees, and gray jays. In the high-elevation meadows you may be fortunate enough to spot violet-green swallows, rufous hummingbirds, red-tailed hawks, mountain bluebirds, Cassin's finches, and horned larks. The alpine areas have the fewest birds, but you may run across gray-crowned rosy finches or white-tailed ptarmigans. Along the park's many rivers and streams you stand a good chance of seeing birds that prefer the watery environment, including American dippers, belted kingfishers, great blue herons, or the rare but quite beautiful harlequin ducks.

Despite an abundance of wonderfully pure and unpolluted water, fish are uncommon at Mount Rainier. Unfortunately, downstream dams have blocked the passage of native steelhead as well as chinook and coho salmon to most of the park's rivers, though these magnificent fish can still sometimes be observed in the Carbon and White river systems. Fish are not native to any of the park's lakes, but stocking has brought several species of trout to these pristine waters. Changes in NPS management policies halted the stocking of fish in 1972, but small, self-sustaining populations of brook, rainbow, and cutthroat trout remain in many lakes. In the rivers and streams not cut off by downstream waterfalls are native populations of coastal cutthroat trout, steelhead, and Dolly Varden and/ or bull trout. In general, the numbers of fish are too small to draw many anglers, and few Wonderland Trail hikers carry fishing equipment.

Though only a small part of the entire wildlife picture, mammals are what most people think of when discussing the animals of Mount Rainier National Park. Only a few mammals are abundant and easily observed. These include small rodents such as Douglas' squirrels and golden-mantled ground squirrels and larger animals such as black-tailed deer, which are often seen in meadows early or late in the day. Like the birds, most mammals are habitat specialists that generally stay within their preferred life zones. The voles, shrews, and other tiny animals that inhabit the forests are rarely seen, but you almost certainly will see Townsend's chipmunks during your hike, and in the evenings it is common to see small bats feasting on insects. If you are very lucky, you may see somewhat larger mammals such as porcupines, snowshoe hares,

Hoary marmot in Moraine Park

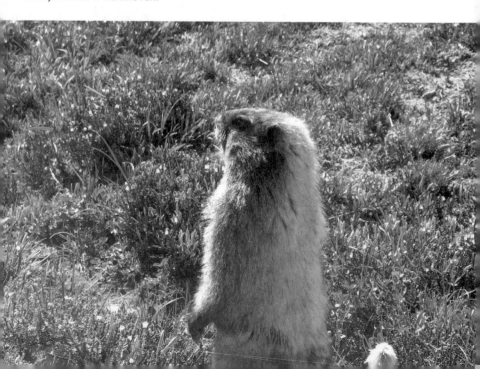

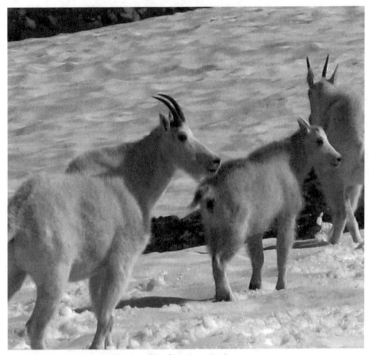

Mountain goats on snowfield south of Panhandle Gap

or pine martens. In rocky areas at higher elevations, look for pikas, shy but exceptionally cute little guinea pig–like animals with rounded ears. They emit a high-pitched "meep" sound that is quite distinctive. Another high-elevation species that you will likely see is the hoary marmot, which is about the size of an overweight house cat. These mammals dig holes in the meadows for their homes and belt out a high whistling sound when alarmed by predators or passing hikers.

Large mammals that inhabit the park include Roosevelt elk (which are most often seen in the meadows in the eastern part of the park), black bears, coyotes, and mountain goats. The last species prefers high-elevation crags, snowfields, and ridges and is most commonly seen by Wonderland Trail hikers on Emerald Ridge, Goat Island Mountain, and Skyscraper

Mountain, and near Panhandle Gap. A partial listing of some of the rarely seen mammals in the park includes river otters, mountain lions, bobcats, northern flying squirrels, and striped skunks.

WEATHER

Apart from a possible illness or injury along the way, nothing will affect your comfort and enjoyment of the Wonderland Trail more than the weather.

As is true throughout the Pacific Northwest, the weather on Mount Rainier is primarily influenced by its proximity to the Pacific Ocean and the string of moisture-laden storms that roll in off that enormous body of water throughout much of the year. During the rainy season, which normally runs about October–May but which occasionally lasts all summer, a seemingly endless series of storms hit the region, usually following a northwest to southeast track. Some of the moisture is extracted by the Olympic Mountains to the west, but there is still plenty of water left by the time the clouds reach the area. The enormous topographic relief of the mountain forces the clouds to climb, and the process progressively squeezes out more precipitation. Thus, at lower elevations on the mountain, the average annual precipitation ranges from "only" 60–80 inches, while at higher elevations that number climbs to 100 inches or more. After passing over the mountain the clouds have lost much of their moisture, which places the east side of Mount Rainier around Sunrise or Summerland in the rain shadow, or more accurately around here the "snow shadow." As a result, these areas are somewhat drier than the west side, though they are still a long way from arid. By the time the storms have made their way over the entire Cascade Range and are passing over central Washington, so much of the water has been extracted that the area is a semidesert with only 15 inches or so of annual precipitation.

During the long winters, the vast majority of precipitation falls as snow, and for a significant percentage of the year all or almost all of Mount Rainier National Park is covered with snow. Fortunately, that is not when you will (or at least should) be hiking the Wonderland Trail. So while it is interesting that Paradise is considered *the snowiest place on Earth* (at least among locations where snow is regularly measured), with a staggering annual average of more than 50 feet, this really affects you only when considering how long into the season it will take for the previous winter's snowpack to melt off the trail.

During the summer months, when rational people hike the trail, the weather is a lot more benign. But that is not to say that you should plan on it being 60–70°F and sunny every day of your hike. In fact, the chances of that happening for the 10–14 days that it takes to complete the trip are just about zero. Even in July and August (generally the best weather months) hail, snow, high winds, fog, blizzards, and especially rain can and do occur, and hikers must be prepared to face these elements. Quality raingear and a good tent are absolute necessities. Attempting the trail without these is a recipe for a great deal of discomfort and possibly disaster. The usual late July or August day on the mountain is partly sunny with a high of 60–75°F, lows in the 40s, and a light breeze or wind, especially at higher elevations. This sounds (and is) very pleasant. Unfortunately, mountain weather in general, and on Mount Rainier in particular, is unpredictable. A clear sky can turn into clouds and rain or even snow in a remarkably short period of time. Check the weather forecasts and watch the skies carefully so you are prepared for what is coming.

Thunderstorms, though not nearly as common on Mount Rainier as they are in places such as the southern Rocky Mountains, should be expected from time to time during the summer. If you see a thunderstorm developing, and especially if you see lightning, do *not* leave the lowlands and climb into the high country. Instead, wait down in the forest for the storm to pass before beginning your ascent. If you find yourself already in the high country when a thunderstorm comes along, then get off that open ridgetop and hightail it back down into forested terrain. Very few areas along the Wonderland Trail remain above timberline for so long that you couldn't simply pick up the pace for a while and find yourself back down in the relative safety of the forest. Typically, thunderstorms last for only an hour or two and then you can resume your trek.

If you are camped at lower elevations during a stretch of good weather in the summer months, especially on the west

Rays of sun through fog near Golden Lakes

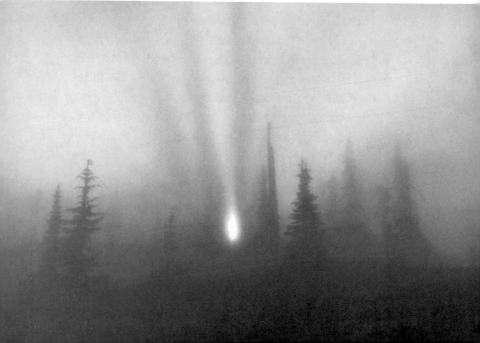

A NOTE ABOUT PHOTOGRAPHY

The good news is that if the weather cooperates, you don't have to be Ansel Adams to take stunning photos while hiking the Wonderland Trail. In fact, much of the time, you'd almost have to be trying *not* to take beautiful pictures. Simply point your camera at the mountain and shoot. The scenery is so outstanding that it's pretty hard to mess things up.

Of course, there are plenty of techniques to help you turn those already good pictures into great ones. Photography books devote hundreds of pages to special lighting techniques, the latest filters, backlighting ideas, and other technical stuff that is really only useful for the advanced photographer. I maintain that the most important thing to do if you want to take beautiful pictures is much more low-tech: go to beautiful places! Fortunately, by hiking the Wonderland Trail, you already have that one covered. So step two is to go to beautiful places *at the right time*. Make a point to climb that ridge above camp as the sun goes down to catch the sunset. Plan your hike so the sun is at your back (not shining directly into the camera lens) when you want to take a picture of the mountain over that classic meadow or lake. Get up early in the morning to catch a mirrorlike reflection in the lake before the wind picks up and ruins things. You get the idea. A little planning will result in much better pictures than if you rely solely on luck.

The next tip is to keep your camera easily accessible. This will allow you to take candid pictures of your hiking companions and obtain that spur-of-the-moment wildlife shot before the animal runs away. Perhaps even more important, having your camera right at hand has a psychological advantage because people whose

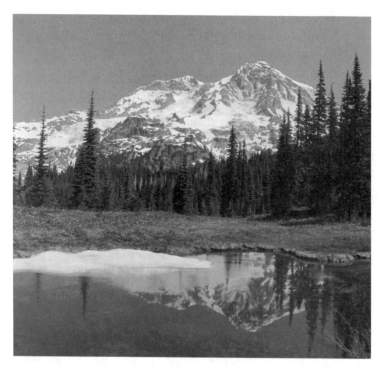

Small pond in Indian Henry's Hunting Ground

photo gear is buried deep in the pack will often talk themselves out of taking what might turn out to be a great picture, just because they don't want to go to the trouble of digging the camera out of its hiding place.

Next, when you have what looks to be a great scene, be sure to take 1) *lots* of pictures (remember, these days it only costs you digital memory; you aren't out a penny for wasted film), 2) pictures from several different angles, and 3) shots that are framed with a tree on the side, flowers in the foreground, interesting clouds in the sky, and so on. These extra elements often make all the difference in the world in the overall quality of your photographs.

One more tip: Because you will undoubtedly be taking lots of pictures, be sure to carry an extra camera battery and a spare memory card. The odds are good that you will need both.

A final very important point about photography involves protecting your equipment. Local weather patterns being what they are, water protection for your camera should be considered a necessity. In addition, with all the rugged terrain along the Wonderland Trail, the occasional fall or bump into a tree is common enough that more than one expensive camera has broken or had its delicate electronic systems damaged. It is important, therefore, that you use good (and tough) camera equipment and protect it in a waterproof case.

side of the mountain near Longmire or along the Carbon or Mowich Rivers, you stand a good chance of waking up beneath a heavy layer of low clouds. This common phenomenon is the result of cool marine air pushing in clouds from Puget Sound and is rarely cause for concern. More often than not, the cloud deck is covering only the lowlands, and once you climb above 3,500 or 4,000 feet you will be in wonderful sunshine. By later in the day the clouds usually burn off, even at lower elevations.

Finally, there is the often-stated fact that Mount Rainier makes its own weather. Because the mountain is so much higher than everything else in the neighborhood, it frequently pokes its nose into the jet stream and gathers clouds around its summit. Thus, it is not uncommon for visitors at lower elevations to be bathed in calm and sunshine while looking up at a mountain (or, more precisely, a cloud bank where the mountain ought to be) where the conditions are very windy and either raining or snowing. Even more common is for hikers to see lenticular clouds, which form over the summit when warm air from the ocean meets the cold of the mountaintop and condenses into clouds. Usually these very photogenic clouds are either mushroom-shaped right over the top of the peak or strung out as high-level winds push them to the east. Lenticular clouds often indicate that the moisture content of the atmosphere is rising and a storm may be on the way.

A Word about Mileages

Hikers who feel the need to know exact mileages are bound to notice something along the Wonderland Trail—you cannot trust the NPS signs. The only thing you can rely on with these signs is that they will be inconsistent. On countless occasions you will be told at one end of a trail that the distance is a specific total, and then upon reaching the other end find a sign telling you that the distance you just covered is actually 0.3 mile or more different. In fairness, part of the problem is that the trail's mileage is constantly in flux. The climate here is very tough on trails. Every year trail crews are forced to reroute sections of the Wonderland Trail to detour around flood damage, washouts, and landslides. In addition, during the high water of spring and early summer, dozens of streams and rivers in the park change their course, forcing seasonal bridges to be moved, slightly altering the trail's total distance.

Many years ago a frustrated guidebook author had a friend get out a measuring wheel and do her own mileage numbers. She was so obsessed with numbers that she even went so far as to tell readers the exact length of every one of the hundreds of bridges along the Wonderland Trail. I am not that extreme, so in doing this book I did not take new measurements, though for maximum accuracy I have generally used the numbers from her book. For new trail sections, or for places where the path has been significantly rerouted, I have used a combination of NPS signs and my own pedometer readings. When I wrote this book, these measurements were as close to accurate as I could reasonably make them. Mother Nature is far from finished with her annual changes, however, so expect the mileages to vary somewhat over time.

That said, despite my training as a certified public accountant, I am not particularly obsessed with mileage numbers and have never seen the functional difference between a distance of, say, 3.9 miles and 4.2 miles. It simply won't change my hiking plans one way or another based on which figure is accurate. Factors such as the elevation gain, trail conditions, my level of tiredness, and the weather all make *far* more difference in hiking time and enjoyment than knowing the mileage down to the nearest tenth. To me the NPS signs are usually close enough. It's mostly a function of attitude. Still, for those of you who just can't live without exact numbers, you will be glad to know that someone at the NPS (who apparently had way too much time on his or her hands) once produced an information sheet telling hikers that the Wonderland Trail (excluding any side trips and the inevitable walking to and around camp) has a total distance of 92.172 miles and a total elevation gain of 22,786 feet. (Unless, of course, you happen to park one or two slots farther away in the parking lot or have to take an extra step around a fallen log, and then your totals will be completely different.)

Opposite: Mount Rainier from pond in Spray Park

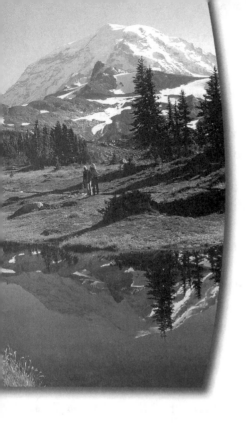

2

Have a Safe (And Fun) Trip

Despite all the bad movies you may have seen about the outdoors, the greatest dangers you are likely to encounter while backpacking are not angry bears, crazy hunters, hungry mountain lions, or "evil" rattlesnakes but more mundane threats such as being wet and cold for too long (which sounds merely uncomfortable but can actually kill you) or falling down and hurting yourself. These concerns might not be "sexy" for the moviemakers, but they are by far the most common types of dangers faced by hikers on the Wonderland Trail, so you need to know how to avoid them to have a safe trip.

Hypothermia

Hypothermia occurs when the body loses more heat than it can produce, thus causing the body's temperature to drop.

When it falls below about 95°F (only 3.6° below normal), hypothermia sets in and symptoms begin to occur (see below). Once your core temperature drops below about 78–80°F, your brain and heart cease to function. People who "freeze to death" actually die of hypothermia long before they freeze.

It does not have to be bitterly cold for a person to suffer from hypothermia. In fact, the overwhelming majority of people who die from hypothermia do so at temperatures *well above* freezing—from 30–50°F is most common, but you can get hypothermia when it is 60°F or more. Typically, people start to feel the effects of hypothermia when they and their clothes are wet from rain or snow and temperatures are in the 40s or 50s. Wind dramatically compounds the problem. Sound familiar? If not, reread the section on "Weather" (beginning on page 21) and you will quickly see why hypothermia is the number one danger to hikers in Mount Rainier National Park. It cannot be stressed enough how important it is that anyone contemplating hiking the Wonderland Trail be equipped with not only the right gear and clothing to avoid hypothermia but also the skills to recognize the symptoms and the knowledge of what to do to reverse it.

Hypothermia can set in remarkably quickly, and because one of the symptoms is a loss of mental functioning and good decision-making skills, you need to regularly monitor both yourself and your companions, so that you can catch the warning signs before your decision-making abilities are impaired. This is particularly crucial if the weather is wet, windy, and cold. The first symptom is shivering, which is your body's attempt to warm itself as its core temperature falls below 95°F. As your temperature continues to fall, you develop signs of confusion and lack of manual dexterity. Once your body's temperature falls below 90°F, you may no longer feel cold but will probably become incoherent and have severe lack of judgment. Things are extremely serious at this point because your body is losing its ability to rewarm itself, and it must receive heat from an outside source. Any further loss of body heat will cause the body to slowly shut down, and you will eventually die. Reversing severe cases of hypothermia can only be done in a medical facility, which is not a realistic option while hiking in the wilderness of Mount Rainier National Park. Therefore, it is very important that mild cases be caught early and treated in the field before they become severe.

You can treat mild cases of hypothermia by getting the affected individual out of the rain and wind as quickly as possible and have him or her move around vigorously. Have the person remove his or her wet clothing and don something dry and warm. If the person is conscious, feed him or her warm liquids, such as hot chocolate or soup, that can be swallowed and digested easily. Place the person in a prewarmed sleeping bag alongside bottles that are filled with warm water. If the hypothermia symptoms are more advanced, have the person strip and place him or her in a warm sleeping bag with one or two other people (also stripped) who curl around the victim and provide skin-to-skin warmth. Despite bad movie advice to the contrary, do *not* give the person alcohol, which will open restricted blood vessels and allow blood to flood the extremities, making the person feel warmer but only at the expense of the body's core, where the warmth is critically needed.

As with most problems, a far better plan than treating cases of hypothermia is to avoid them in the first place. The best way to do this is to wear adequate clothing and to try to avoid potentially dangerous situations, such as hiking for prolonged periods along exposed ridges when the weather is cold, windy, and raining or snowing. As previously mentioned, you absolutely *must* carry good raingear that will protect both you and the clothes worn beneath your raingear from getting wet. The raingear should also be made from material that serves as an effective shield against the wind. After good boots, a quality rain jacket is probably the single most important item that you will carry on your trip around the mountain. Rain pants may also help to protect your lower body. Without them, your legs will get absolutely soaked, if not from the rain itself then from all the water that collects on plants that you brush up against while hiking. A warm knit pullover cap is also a requirement because an enormous amount of your body's heat is lost through your head. In clear and cool weather the knit cap will also make evenings around camp much more comfortable and keep your head toasty while you are sleeping.

In addition to the right clothing, you should keep your body well hydrated and, most important, well fed. At regular intervals refuel with high-energy foods, such as energy bars, nuts, and candy, which provide quick calories for your body to burn and warm up. Have these foods easily accessible, so you don't have to stop to dig them out of your pack. When you stop to rest, do so out of the wind and cover up as quickly as possible because your body will rapidly cool down once you stop hiking.

Accidents

As the old saying goes, accidents happen. And despite what your ego and emotions would like to believe, they can and do happen to you. Even the most experienced and best-conditioned hikers sometimes lose their concentration, step on a loose rock or icy patch, and find themselves either flat on their backside or, much worse, tumbling down a brush- or rock-covered slope. The rugged terrain along the Wonderland Trail is not only spectacularly scenic but also potentially hazardous. Badly twisted ankles and knees, broken bones, and severe cuts are just a few of the accident-related injuries that strike Wonderland Trail hikers every year. Most of the time these result in nothing worse than a lot of discomfort and a ruined trip, but occasionally they can be a threat not only to your vacation plans and ego but also to your life.

I realize that this is going to sound simplistic, but the best way to avoid falling and injuring yourself is to use common sense and not do anything that overextends your body or that a disinterested observer might uncharitably describe as "stupid." Before you cross a raging stream by walking over that slippery log, scramble out to that dangerously exposed point merely to get a slightly better picture, or step on that wobbly boulder without checking its stability first, remember that a hospital or, for that matter, any kind of trained medical assistance is a long way (and, more important, a long *time*) away. It is also worth remembering that despite what your ego would like to believe, you probably aren't 18 anymore and your body more than likely is not as strong and limber as it used to be. Unfortunately, clear thinking like this becomes increasingly difficult when you are tired at the end of a long day on the trail.

Here are a few tips to avoid getting into accidents while on the trail:

1) Develop the habit of taking a deep breath and considering things before doing *anything* that could be dangerous. Initially this will seem a bit ridiculous and probably feel like overkill, but eventually it will become second nature and could save your life.

2) Take regular rest stops, both to refresh your body and to keep your mind sharp. This is easy to do on long uphills

because physical exhaustion will require that you take a breather. What far too many people forget to do, however, is to also take rest stops on longer *downhills*. People don't feel winded so they figure that they don't need a breather. Your knees and toes will greatly appreciate it, however, and, at least as important, your mind will have a chance to recharge and be more careful about foot placement and other safety issues.

3)   Avoid cross-country travel unless weather conditions allow for easy navigation, you are experienced in off-trail hiking, and the terrain is safe for travel.

4)   Be especially careful when crossing steep snowfields or anywhere that ice has formed on the trail—a frequent occurrence because mornings can be frosty in the mountains at any time of year.

5)   When hiking downhill, take short, measured steps and watch carefully for hazards such as ice, mud, wet rocks, roots, and loose gravel. It is also a good idea to use a hiking staff or pole (some people use two) to help with your stability.

6)   Finally, plan your trip to avoid long descents at the end of the day when you are probably going to be tired and are more likely to make mistakes.

Blisters, Aches and Pains, and Injuries

I was once asked to give a presentation to a group of beginning backpackers. It took me a while to determine how best to begin my speech, but deciding that honesty was the best policy, I figured it was best to start out with the truth. So I told the eager group of young people that backpacking has the potential to open up a wonderful world of solitude, challenge, and spectacular scenery, but perhaps the first and most important thing that a novice needs to know about backpacking is . . . that it hurts! I informed my now startled audience that more than likely, they would get sore muscles, itchy mosquito bites, and perhaps a blister or two, and for much of the time they would feel uncomfortable. But, I then made sure to say, nothing truly worthwhile in life comes easily. If it did, we wouldn't value it. Heck, I pointed out, playing any of the sports that so many people enjoy requires lots of effort and probably many of the same sore muscles and blisters (though, I had to concede, mosquito bites aren't usually considered a significant hazard for the typical, say, volleyball player).

Well, I had their attention by then, and I hope, especially if you are new to backpacking, I have yours as well. Backpacking in general, and the Wonderland Trail in particular, involves

Backpacker on Emerald Ridge

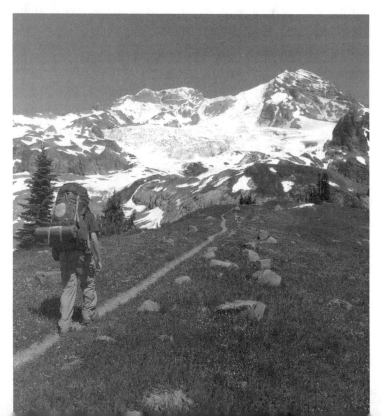

considerable effort and some sacrifice. One potential sacrifice is your comfort. Still, the whole point of this exercise is not just, well, exercise but also to have a good time. It's not a death march, after all; it's a vacation. So here I will discuss a few reasonable measures that you can take to make your trek as comfortable as possible.

The best way to avoid blisters, which can be nearly debilitating, is to wear boots that fit comfortably and are well broken in. Do not under any circumstances start out on a trip as demanding as the Wonderland Trail in a brand-new pair of boots. While it is true that boots today are significantly better than the heavy wafflestompers that we tramped around in decades ago, they still require some fine-tuning to get the right fit. Take several day hikes and shorter backpacking trips with your new footwear to see how it does when you are carrying a heavy load on rough trails. Fine-tune the fit with one or two pairs of high-quality hiking socks, making especially sure to eliminate any rubbing on your sensitive toes and heels. Also, replace the factory-made insoles with something of higher quality. Finally, be careful to make sure that the boots are waterproof, either by having Gore-Tex or another similar material in the boots themselves or by waterproofing the leather. Keeping your feet dry and comfortable should solve virtually all of the blister issues and make your trip infinitely more enjoyable. If, despite all this stellar advice, your boots still start to rub you the wrong way, then *stop hiking* while the hot spot on your foot is still only a hot spot and not already a blister. Cover the tender area with athletic tape or Moleskin. This will help prevent a blister from forming. Continue to cover the same location every morning as a preventive measure. If you develop a blister anyway, then cover it with blister tape or surround it with a raised doughnut of Moleskin, and then cover both the blister and the Moleskin with athletic tape.

Backpackers frequently suffer from a variety of general aches and pains. These occur most frequently on tender hips and shoulders that are unaccustomed to carrying a pack. Such aches and pains are usually less troublesome than blisters, but they are not necessarily less painful. Again, the best plan is to stop these in their tracks before they become major problems. Make sure that your backpack fits well and is adjusted properly for both your body shape and the amount of weight you will be carrying. A good salesperson at the outdoors store where you purchase the pack can be helpful here. As with boots, do not set out on the Wonderland Trail in a brand-new pack that you have not yet taken on shorter trips, which allow you to work out the kinks and get the best fit. Beyond that, about all you can do on the trail is to provide yourself with some extra jury-rigged padding by stuffing socks or the like under your shoulder straps. Not ideal, but it's better than nothing.

Sore muscles are common, especially for people who do not backpack regularly and who are suddenly using muscles that have remained idle when doing other activities. Plenty of stretching both in the morning and in the evening, a good night's sleep, and a vigorous massage (either a self-massage or, much more fun, one that is performed by a willing partner) will help a lot. You should also carry over-the-counter painkillers such as ibuprofen or aspirin to help with these low-level discomfort issues.

More difficult problems arise when you get seriously injured on the trail. Knees and ankles are especially vulnerable and frequently suffer from sprains, severe twists, and even breaks. (Personally, I think these "weak" body parts are the result of a design flaw, but I am unwilling to take this up with the designer Himself lest I appear ungrateful.) These sorts of injuries are especially troublesome because they will quickly bring your trip to a crashing halt. Long, steep downhills, of which the

Wonderland Trail has more than its share, are especially tough on knees. The best plan is to walk slowly, take short strides, use trekking poles, and try to avoid long downhills late in the day when you are tired, less stable, and more prone to falls. People with known knee issues should consider wearing a knee brace. If you do twist your knee or ankle, then stop immediately, take anti-inflammatory drugs such as ibuprofen or naproxen, and wrap the joint using an elastic bandage (if it is a knee) or athletic tape (if it is an ankle). Following this treatment, you can usually continue *slowly* hiking using trekking poles or a companion as improvised crutches. At the next available opportunity, exit the trail and stop your hike. Completing the Wonderland Trail that year is not in the cards.

Bears, Bugs, and Other Critters

Mount Rainier National Park has a healthy population of American black bears, and if you hike the entire Wonderland Trail, you stand a better than even chance of seeing one (or more) along the way. These bears are particularly active at night, when they engage in their favorite pursuit: searching for food. In this capacity, they happily resort to the role of large, hairy thief bent on stealing any not-carefully-enough-protected offerings. When camping in one of the park's designated backcountry campsites, you should hang your food, and anything else that may smell enticing, on the food pole or wire provided at that camp. This will protect your precious supplies not only from the bruins but also from another common thief: chipmunks. As for the possibility of bear attacks, these are so rare that they really aren't worth worrying about. Still, it is always wise to avoid bears, and especially to never get between a sow and her cubs.

A far more common wildlife problem comes from mosquitoes. These nasty little vampires bite, buzz, and are generally very annoying from shortly after snowmelt through about mid-August. Come prepared to deal with the insect infidels by carrying repellent, wearing long-sleeve shirts and long pants, using a tent with mosquito netting, and employing lots of either patience or swear words, depending on your personality. These strategies also work against flies, which can sometimes present a problem on warm days in late summer. Finally, ticks are rare but are sometimes seen at lower elevations in the northwest part of the park. To date, these ticks have not been found to carry diseases such as Lyme disease or Rocky Mountain spotted fever. If you check yourself regularly and pull the disgusting little buggers out as soon as you find them, then you should be fine.

As for other wildlife that hikers sometimes worry about, such as snakes, grizzly bears, mountain lions, and the like, forget about them. Mount Rainier National Park has no poisonous snakes, and the small garter snakes that do live here are harmless and actually rather cute. Grizzly bears do not live in

A black bear walking through Sunset Park

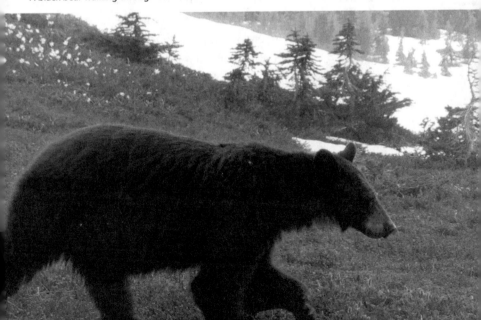

the park, and while mountain lions are fairly common, they are almost never seen and present no real danger to human beings (there hasn't been a reported attack by a mountain lion in the history of the park).

Other Safety Issues

WATER PURIFICATION

Although the water in the lakes and streams of Mount Rainier National Park may look pure, hikers should *never drink water from any natural source without purifying it first.* Nasty little microorganisms, in particular a parasite called giardia, may live in these waters and have the ability to cause all kinds of miserable symptoms (nausea, severe weakness, headaches, and projectiles from pretty much every orifice), which will, at a minimum, ruin your trip. It's just not worth the gamble. Purify *all* water by boiling it (inconvenient and uses lots of fuel), chemically treating it, or filtering it before consumption. A newer method involves using an ultraviolet light stick, which generally works well on giardia but does not remove particulate matter. It is also strongly advised that you not drink the heavily silt-laden water that comes from the many glacial streams on Mount Rainier. In an emergency, you *could* purify the water by letting it settle in a pot for several minutes and then filtering it, but there is generally no need to do this. In this wet environment a nice, clear creek is almost always a reasonable distance away and would be a much better water source.

BRIDGES

All of the rivers and most of the lesser creeks you encounter along the Wonderland Trail have bridges across them for the convenience and safety of hikers. However, these waterways have a disturbing tendency to flood and sometimes to simply change course, either wiping out that convenient bridge or leaving it high and dry. In addition, some of the bridges are nothing but temporary log structures that are installed as conditions permit early in the hiking season and then removed shortly before the snow starts to fall. When you pick up your permit, always ask about the status of bridges along the trail. If an important bridge has been washed out, the trail may be closed until a new bridge can be put in place.

CROSSING STREAMS

As the snow melts early in the season, the streams rampage down their canyons, occasionally swamping the bridges and requiring you to ford the river. In addition, some of the lesser creeks, which may not have a bridge at all, occasionally present hazards during the high runoff period of early summer. Be extremely careful when faced with this situation. If a stream is more than knee deep, if it is swift (pretty much all the streams here are swift), and especially if it is a glacial stream so full of silt that you cannot see the bottom, then *do not try to cross*

Log bridge over North Mowich River

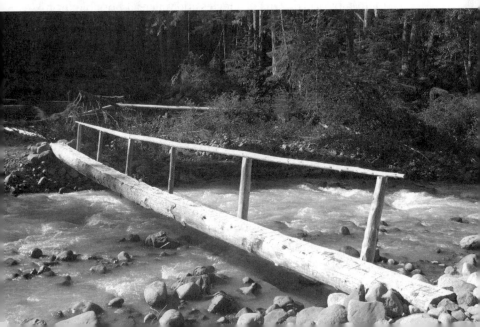

it. It's just too dangerous. Turn around and head back to the nearest trailhead. If you must cross a stream, remember that the volume of water can dramatically change with the time of day. On warm summer days the melting of snow and ice in the afternoon will add considerably to the flow. As a result, always try to cross streams early in the morning, when the water level is typically lower.

GLACIERS

Glaciers present a special hazard on Mount Rainier because they are sometimes right beside the trail, and their deep crevasses, sudden movements of ice, and often unstable and rocky banks can be extremely dangerous for people who venture onto or near them. Unless you are properly outfitted with climbing gear and have advanced climbing skills, then *stay the heck off any glacier*! Usually this is required by park regulations, and it's certainly required by common sense.

MUSHROOMS

Mushrooms are a Pacific Northwest specialty. The damp climate supports dozens of species and makes it possible for hikers to find mushrooms in any season—late August–November is usually best. In Mount Rainier National Park the fungi are most common in dense old-growth forests at lower elevations. Unlike edible berries, which the park allows hikers to pick in small amounts for personal consumption, collecting mushrooms in any quantity is prohibited. The reason for this ban is to protect the mushrooms as an important part of the ecosystem, but there is also a safety issue. Several poisonous species grow in the park, and it is often difficult to tell them apart. Some people have become seriously ill after making a mistake in identification. It is much better to simply enjoy these interesting and often colorful fungi with your eyes instead of your tongue. In any event, you'll be carrying several pounds of food that you are sure is safe, and if only to reduce your pack weight, you are better off eating that instead of the possibly dangerous local flora.

GEOLOGICAL DISASTERS

Guidebooks almost never mention the potential dangers from geologic events such as volcanic eruptions or earthquakes simply because the chances of such things happening are so remote that it just isn't worth the reader's time. On Mount Rainier, however, that is not quite true. While the odds of an eruption happening during your visit are extremely small, the chances of less dramatic but no less dangerous events such as mudflows or debris flows, while still unlikely, are high enough

Shelf fungus on tree near South Mowich River

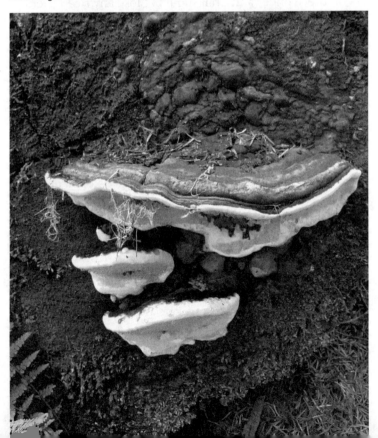

that at least a few words are warranted. Lahars (volcanic mudflows), for example, happen with disturbing regularity on Mount Rainier, especially in certain glacial-stream canyons on the west side of the mountain. In the 1980s and 1990s on Tahoma Creek, for example, lahars seemed to be happening all the time. Four separate flows occurred in 1989 alone. The Nisqually River and Kautz Creek have also been quite active in recent times, with the enormous flow in October 1947 on Kautz Creek being particularly noteworthy. It is certainly possible that a lahar could occur again on any of the glacial canyons of Mount Rainier. As mentioned in the "Geology" section beginning on page 8, devastating debris flows have also occurred in recent times on the White River. Interestingly, these events are not necessarily tied to volcanic activity or to major earthquakes. They just seem to happen. So while hikers on the Wonderland Trail shouldn't lose any sleep over the possibility of a lahar or debris flow overwhelming them on their trek, they should at least know what to do if one occurs. The best advice for anyone camping in or traveling through a glacial valley is to stay alert and watch for signs of trouble. If you hear a loud, rumbling, freight train–like sound; feel a blast of air rushing down the canyon; notice a violent trembling in the ground; or see the water level in the river or creek rising rapidly, then *get to higher ground immediately*. Statistics show that you may have only one or two minutes before a debris or mudflow arrives. Generally, climbing just 150 feet in elevation should put you out of any immediate danger.

CRIME

Unfortunately, even national parks are not immune from the world's criminal element, so hikers need to take reasonable steps to protect their property. It is very rare for items to be stolen from backcountry campsites (thieves have to carry the loot out and must work too hard for any potential gains), but if you leave your camp unattended for a significant length of time, it's always wise to take your wallet, camera, and other small and valuable items with you. A more common problem is car break-ins. Although relatively infrequent at Mount Rainier National Park, break-ins do occur, and backpackers, who necessarily leave their vehicles unattended for several days in a row, are more likely to encounter this problem than day hikers. Do not encourage the criminals by providing unnecessary temptation. Preferably, leave the new car at home and drive an older, beat-up vehicle instead. Unfortunately, this is generally not an option for out-of-state hikers who have flown into Seattle and rented a car. In this case, about all you can do is to avoid renting one of the top-end, expensive models. Most important, leave nothing of value inside your car, especially not in plain sight. My car has been broken into three times over the years (though not at Mount Rainier, yet). The last two times, all the thieves managed to take home were some ratty old tennis shoes. If all trailhead vehicles held items of similar value, the criminals would soon give up.

ALTITUDE SICKNESS

Hikers familiar with the problems of altitude sickness in other popular hiking areas around the American West, such as California's Sierra Nevada or the Colorado Rockies, will be glad to know that there are virtually no such problems on the Wonderland Trail. The entire trail is below 6,800 feet, so the air never gets too thin even for people who live near sea level. For the first day or two you may notice a bit of extra wheezing due to a marginal decrease in the oxygen content of the air (assuming, that is, you could distinguish this wheezing from that brought on by the steep grades and rough terrain), but there is no reason to worry about the more uncomfortable or even dangerous effects of altitude sickness, such as loss of appetite, nausea, dizziness, severe headaches, and shortness of breath.

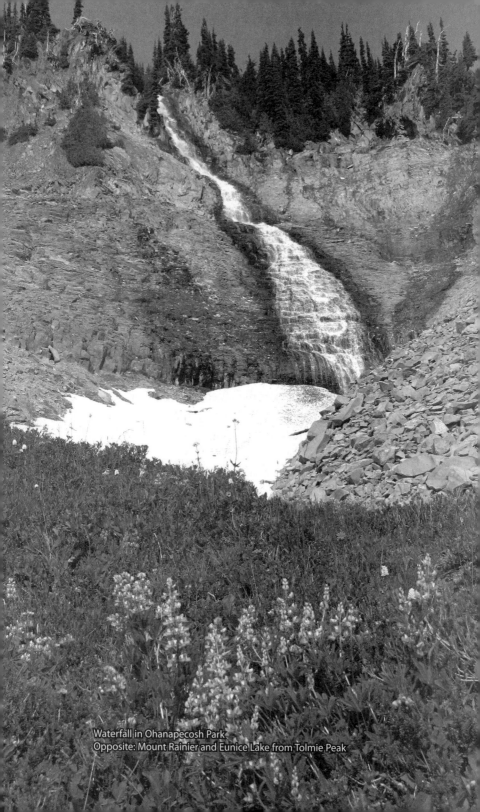

Waterfall in Ohanapecosh Park
Opposite: Mount Rainier and Eunice Lake from Tolmie Peak

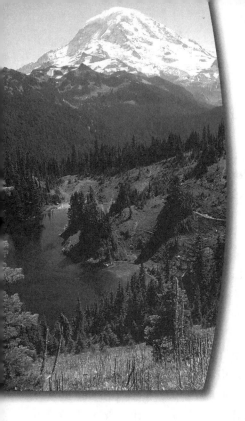

3

Planning and Preparation

OK, so you've read all the glowing reports in this book and elsewhere and are understandably excited about doing the Wonderland Trail. Now it's time for some careful planning and a sober assessment of your abilities to make sure that you can do the trip safely, reasonably comfortably, and in a way that affords maximum enjoyment.

Section Hikes or All at Once?

One of the first questions to ask yourself is whether you have the time and physical ability to do the entire trip. Certainly the *best* way to see the mountain and enjoy everything the magnificent park has to offer is to take the entire Wonderland Trail in one grand adventure. For a variety of reasons, however, that's not always possible.

For most reasonably fit hikers the complete Wonderland Trail takes a minimum of 8–10 days, and often up to 13–14 days when you include extra time for side trips and possible layover days. While the trail is unquestionably worth every minute, that is still a significant chunk out of most people's vacation time. In addition, even those who have that kind of time could still conclude that their knees, shoulders, feet, and other assorted body parts would feel considerably better about the world if the overly enthusiastic brain didn't commit them to something they just aren't up for. The best plan is to hold a vote. If any of the various body parts casts a firm "no" vote, consider it a veto on the entire operation. Consensus here is crucial to avoid the unfortunate circumstance where the reluctant voter ends up refusing to participate halfway through your adventure, which creates real problems for all concerned. When holding the vote, it is important that no one part gets pressured into voting "yes" when it really should be voting "no." In other words, be brutally honest about your physical limitations and conditioning. Remember that in any given year tens of thousands of people hike parts of the Wonderland Trail, but only about 200–250 people complete the entire trip. You're in good company.

Fortunately, deciding that the full loop is too much for your body or your vacation budget does not mean that you can't enjoy the countless wonders of the Wonderland Trail. The trail breaks up nicely into segments that, while still challenging, are easier to tackle than the whole kit and caboodle. Chapter 4 breaks the trail up into logical segments that work well for people doing the hike piecemeal. Also several excellent sections of the trail can be done in as little as a day. For hikers who don't like the idea of returning on the same trail they hiked in on, there are several loops that combine the Wonderland with alternate trails. What follows are my recommendations for the best shorter options for exploring the Wonderland Trail, depending on the amount of time you have available.

Best Day Hikes:

1) Spray Park and ridge from Mowich Lake (8.2 miles round-trip)

2) Longmire (upper trailhead) to the end of the Westside Road via Indian Henry's Hunting Ground and Tahoma Creek (11.6 miles one way—a car shuttle is required and the Tahoma Creek Trail is quite rough, so it should be taken only by experienced hikers)

3) Berkeley Park and Skyscraper Pass from Sunrise (7-plus miles round-trip)

4) Ohanapecosh Falls from the Deer Creek Trailhead on Washington Highway 123 (6.8 miles round-trip—actually on the Eastside alternative to the Wonderland Trail, but perfect for a cloudy day)

Best Weekend Backpacking Trips:

1) Ipsut Pass, Carbon River, Seattle Park, and Spray Park from Mowich Lake (16.4-mile loop)

2) White River Road to Box Canyon via Panhandle Gap (16.4 miles one way—a car shuttle is required)

3) Box Canyon to Indian Bar (15.2 miles round-trip)

Best 3- to 4-Day Backpacking Trips:

1) Wonderland Trail—Northern Loop Trail loop from Sunrise via Berkeley Park, Mystic Lake, Carbon River, Windy Gap, Lake James, and Grand Park (33.4-mile loop)

2)   Wonderland Trail—Eastside Trail loop from White River via Owyhigh Lakes, Ohanapecosh River, Cowlitz Divide, Indian Bar, and Summerland (33.6-mile loop)

3)   Longmire (upper trailhead) to Mowich Lake (33.8 miles one way—a *long* car shuttle is required)

When to Go

When should you hike the Wonderland Trail? The short answer is summer, and preferably you should narrow that down to mid- to late summer or perhaps early fall. People occasionally inquire about winter travel on the trail, but unless you are a very experienced cold-weather wilderness expert, it cannot be stressed enough how difficult and dangerous taking the Wonderland Trail in winter would be. The weather is frequently awful (think almost constant cloud cover, cold temperatures, and frequent whiteout conditions), navigation is extremely difficult, and the chance of a rescue should anything happen to you is next to impossible. Put simply: Forget about it.

Spring—which is defined at these latitudes and altitudes as from about May to early July—and mid- to late fall (late September–November) are also pretty wet, and in spring you must contend with a trail that remains encased in several feet of snow. The first significant snowfall of the season usually happens in early to mid-October.

So that leaves a realistic window of opportunity for doing the Wonderland Trail from about mid-July–mid-September. Within that rather short two-month period, however, the conditions vary dramatically. In a typical year, hikers in mid-July should expect a fair amount of lingering snow, especially at higher elevations around Klapatche Park, Spray Park, and Panhandle Gap. In addition, streams will be full of snowmelt, and many portions of the trail will be muddy. On the other hand, the wildflower displays at midelevations can be outstanding, and the number of backpackers has not yet hit its peak, so obtaining a permit is usually a little easier. If your research shows that the previous winter's snowpack was significantly below normal, then mid-July would be an excellent time to do the trip.

Late July–mid-August is probably prime time to do the hike. The weather (at least on average) is at its best, the wildflowers in the high meadows are peaking, most of the snow is off the trail, and the scenery is terrific. On the other hand, a lot of people agree with everything I just wrote, so demand for permits is at its highest, and to get one you will probably have to settle for campsites that you did not initially prefer or have in mind. Mosquitoes are also a problem at this time of year, so be prepared.

Late August and early September can be an outstanding time to take the Wonderland Trail. The bugs are mostly gone, the trails are in excellent condition (maintenance is complete and the tread is usually dry), and there is slightly less demand for permits. Unfortunately, most of the flowers will be past their peak and the weather gets progressively cooler and iffier the later you go.

In mid- to late September conditions can be wonderful—no bugs, relatively few people, some fall colors starting in the high country, easily obtained permits, and well-maintained trails—but the big downside is that the weather can be very touch and go. Snow is a distinct possibility, and at least some rain is virtually guaranteed. I am sure that it is theoretically possible to complete the Wonderland Trail in the latter part of September under beautiful weather with continuously sunny skies, but it is probably more likely that hikers will find themselves slogging through rain for almost the entire trip. If that prospect deters you, then either try another time of year or start praying to the weather gods.

Despite everything written above, in really heavy snow years, large portions of the trail may never be free of snow, making hiking the trail at any time difficult and sometimes dangerous. You can mitigate things somewhat by taking the lower-elevation alternate routes on the north and east sides of the mountain (see trail descriptions), but even this may not completely eliminate the problem. In this case, the only realistic alternatives are to either try another year or give it a go anyway but be sure to wear good waterproof boots, have better-than-average navigation skills, bring glacier glasses to protect your eyes from snow glare, and be prepared to do a bit of postholing to cross some snowfields.

One of the first things you should do before planning your vacation and sending in your permit application is to check that year's snowpack to see how it compares to normal. The easiest way to do this is to check the National Resource Conservation Service's website at **www.wa.nrcs.usda.gov/snow.** If the data show that Mount Rainier's snowpack as of March (when you will be sending in your reservation application) is significantly above or below normal, then adjust your travel plans accordingly.

Where to Start

The majority of people who do the Wonderland Trail loop begin at Longmire, on the southwest side of the mountain. The choice is reasonable because Longmire is conveniently located, a wilderness information center is just 75 yards from the trailhead, and there is plenty of parking. In deference to tradition, this book's trail description begins at Longmire and goes in the also-traditional clockwise fashion.

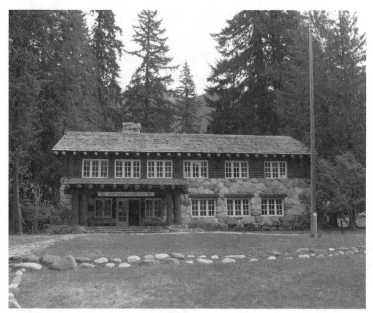

Longmire Wilderness Information Center

But the most popular way to do something is not necessarily the *best* way to do something. There are several other possible starting points, and which one you use will depend on how easy it is to get a permit, the timing and spacing of food caches, what kind of shape you are in at the start of the trip, and a host of other factors. Some of the advantages and disadvantages of the various starting point options are discussed below.

Mowich Lake, in the northwest part of the park, is my favorite starting point for the Wonderland Trail. Beginning here makes your first day or two easier than if you started at Longmire, especially if you plan to take the official Wonderland Trail instead of the more popular Spray Park Trail alternative from Mowich Lake. Thus, while your pack weight is at its greatest, you can gradually get yourself into hiking shape as you go along. On the other hand, the access road into Mowich Lake is gravel and rather bumpy, so some people might not want to drive it, particularly if they just rented a car at the Seattle-Tacoma International Airport. More important, the process of obtaining a backcountry permit is more cumbersome when starting at Mowich Lake because there is no wilderness information center here. To pick up your permit you must drive an extra 16 miles round-trip to the Carbon River Ranger Station, which is located at the end of Carbon River Road near the northwest corner of the park. In 2011 (hours change from year to year) that facility had summer hours 8:30 a.m.–5 p.m. Monday–Thursday and 7:30 a.m.–7 p.m. Friday–Sunday, so it generally opens later than the Longmire Wilderness Information Center. This puts you at a disadvantage if you are trying to obtain a first-come, first-serve permit because others may have used that extra time to grab all the available camping spots. In addition, the Carbon River Ranger Station is still at least an hour's drive from the Mowich Lake Trailhead, so you won't be able to get as early a start on your first day.

The next reasonable starting locations for the Wonderland Trail are all reachable from White River Road in the northeast section of the park: Sunrise, the White River Campground, and the Fryingpan Creek/Summerland Trailhead. These have the advantage of good road access, and you pass the White River Wilderness Information Center on the drive in, so it is easy to pick up your permit and check on the latest trail and weather conditions. If you are taking the trail clockwise, starting at Sunrise forces you into a very long first day before you reach the first allowable backpacker campsite at Summerland. Thus, most people who start at Sunrise do the trail in the marginally less desirable counterclockwise fashion. Starting at either White River Campground or the Summerland Trailhead has no significant downsides except that if you are beginning your hike on a weekend, it can be extremely difficult to obtain an unreserved permit for the very popular Summerland campsite. Also, the Fryingpan Creek/Summerland Trailhead has very limited parking, which makes it better for hikers who are just being dropped off.

The final logical starting point is at Box Canyon along the Stevens Canyon Road (also known as Washington Highway 706) in the southeast part of the park. By starting here you will hike the marginally less scenic southern section of the Wonderland Trail first and, as a result, save the best scenery for last. This location is less convenient to wilderness information centers, however, and parking is somewhat limited.

You can also start at other locations such as the Reflection Lakes or the Westside Road, but the spacing of campsites and/ or longer access trails make these options less appealing.

How Long to Take

Once you have decided to do the entire Wonderland Trail, instead of one of the shorter section hikes or loops discussed above, then you must come up with a reasonable itinerary. The number of possible itineraries is almost limitless depending on where you decide to start, how far you want to travel each day, the number of side trips you plan to take, the vacation time you have available, what kind of hiking shape you are in, where you plan for food caches, the number of layover days (if any) you want to take, and countless other factors. In 2003 a runner reportedly completed the trail in just over 24 hours, but if we restrict ourselves to a sane schedule, then the usual itinerary involves a total of 8–13 days.

Two sample itineraries, both starting at Longmire, are shown below. Both itineraries include the tougher, more scenic, and more popular Spray Park alternative to the Wonderland

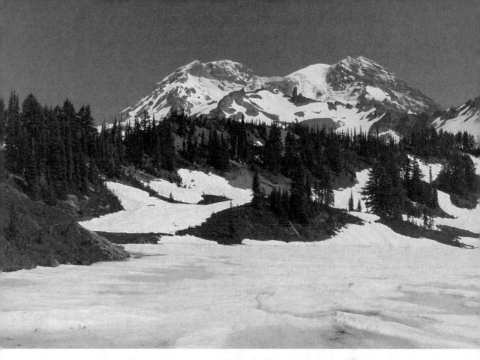

Mount Rainier over frozen St. Andrews Lake

Trail. The first itinerary is shorter and would be better for well-conditioned hikers who have a restricted time frame for completing the trail. The second is a longer itinerary for hikers who prefer a more leisurely pace and/or want to take more side trips. As mentioned above there are innumerable other options, but these should give you a good starting point in your planning.

Shorter 9-Day Sample Itinerary:

Day 1: Longmire to Devil's Dream Camp (5.9 miles)

Day 2: Devil's Dream Camp to North Puyallup River Camp (13.2 miles)

Day 3: North Puyallup River Camp to South Mowich River Camp (10.9 miles)

Day 4: South Mowich River Camp to Cataract Valley Camp (10.4 miles), plus side trips to Spray Falls and Upper Spray Park

Day 5: Cataract Valley Camp to Mystic Camp (6.9 miles), plus a side trip to Willis Wall viewpoint

Day 6: Mystic Camp to Sunrise Camp (8.7 miles), plus a side trip to Sunrise Lodge to pick up your food cache

Day 7: Sunrise Camp to Summerland Camp (9.9 miles)

Day 8: Summerland Camp to Nickel Creek Camp (11.3 miles)

Day 9: Nickel Creek Camp to Longmire (13.9 miles)

Longer 12-Day Sample Itinerary:

Day 1: Longmire to Devil's Dream Camp (5.9 miles)

Day 2: Devil's Dream Camp to Klapatche Park (10.4 miles), plus side trips to Mirror Lakes and Aurora Peak

Day 3: Klapatche Park to Golden Lakes (7.8 miles), plus a side trip to the Sunset Park viewpoint

Day 4: Golden Lakes to Mowich Lake (10 miles), with a food cache pickup at Mowich Lake

Day 5: Mowich Lake to Cataract Valley Camp (6.7 miles), plus side trips to Spray Falls, around Spray Park, and Upper Spray Park

Day 6: Cataract Valley Camp to Mystic Camp (6.9 miles)

Day 7: Layover day at Mystic Camp (0 miles); possible day hike side trip to Willis Wall viewpoint

Day 8: Mystic Camp to Sunrise Camp (8.7 miles)

Day 9: Sunrise Camp to Summerland Camp (9.9 miles), with a food cache pickup at White River Campground

Day 10: Summerland Camp to Indian Bar (4.5 miles), plus a side trip to buttes above Panhandle Gap

Day 11: Indian Bar to Maple Creek Camp (10 miles)

Day 12: Maple Creek Camp to Longmire (10.7 miles)

Note: Keep in mind that it is possible (even likely) that you will be forced into a somewhat different itinerary than what you originally planned. Rangers must frequently give out permits that include alternate campsites because other hikers have already reserved all the available space at your preferred site. Don't be overly disappointed by this. After all, there really are no bad itineraries when the entire trail is so outstanding.

Once on the trail, making changes to your campsite locations is usually impossible.

What to Bring

Probably more pages in backpacking how-to books are devoted to gear than any other single topic. It can get rather overwhelming, and if you aren't careful, it can also get pretty expensive. Remember that despite what it may seem like when shopping at the outdoors store, it is certainly possible (even preferable) to do the Wonderland Trail without breaking into your 401(k) account and taking out a second mortgage on the house. There are only a few items where the extra expense is critical. Beyond that, stick with the basics and you should be fine.

THE TEN ESSENTIALS

Long experience in the backcountry has shown that every hiker should carry a few critical items that have been termed the ten essentials. These should *always* be with you whether you are backpacking, day hiking, or just taking a short side trip. *Never* leave them behind. The standard ten essentials have evolved from a list of individual items into functional systems that will help to keep you alive and reasonably comfortable in emergency situations.

1. *Navigation:* a topographic map and a compass or GPS device
2. *Sun protection:* sunglasses and sunscreen
3. *Insulation:* extra clothing that is both waterproof and warm
4. *Illumination:* a flashlight or headlamp
5. First-aid supplies
6. *Fire:* a candle or other fire starter and matches in a waterproof container
7. *Repair kit:* particularly a knife for starting fires, first aid, and countless other uses
8. *Nutrition:* enough extra food so you return with a little left over

9. *Hydration:* extra water and a means to purify more on longer trips

10. *Emergency shelter:* a tent, bivy sack, or emergency blanket

I strongly advise adding a small plastic signaling whistle and a warm knit cap to the list.

Just carrying these items, however, does not make you prepared. Unless you know how to apply basic first aid, how to build an emergency fire, and how to read a topographic map or use a compass, carrying these items does you no good. These skills are all fairly simple, and at least one member of your group should be familiar with each of them.

THE BASIC GEAR

Beyond the 10 essentials, the tricky part about deciding what to carry on your trip around Mount Rainier is the constant balancing act between comfort and safety on one side and weight on the other. Some items are no-brainers in that you really have no choice about carrying, for example, a sleeping bag, a rain jacket, or a first-aid kit. But things aren't quite that simple because even the no-brainers involve choices about what kind of sleeping bag to carry (down versus synthetic fill), the type of rain jacket to bring along (a simple plastic covering or a high-quality Gore-Tex shell), and just how much stuff to pack into your first-aid kit. The basic rule of thumb is to always look for ways to reduce your pack weight without overly compromising your comfort or safety. If it is a close call between comfort and weight, you should generally opt for less weight because the lower weight will also improve your comfort. When it is a choice between safety and weight, then go for safety because the risk just isn't worth the reduction in ounces.

Later in this section are three complete lists: first of those, items you *must* take; second, of optional items you should consider taking; and finally, of things people sometimes take

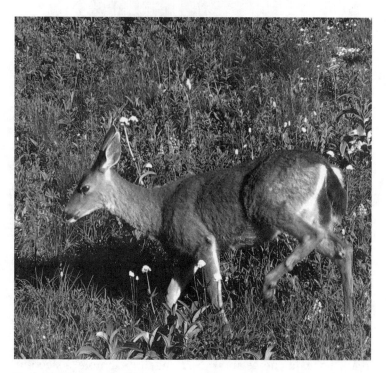

Black-tailed doe near Mystic Lake

but should probably leave behind. For now, I will discuss in detail only a few of the more important items you will be lugging around, make some recommendations, and show you how to tailor your gear to the unique needs and demands of the Wonderland Trail. Not all the items you will be carrying are covered here. Items not requiring further commentary are simply shown on the lists.

Item one of the required gear is something in which to carry all the other items: a **backpack.** This does not have to be a fancy new model costing several hundred dollars. After all, thousands of people have done the Wonderland Trail in old packs with frayed edges and many hundreds of trail miles already on their slightly dented frames. What *is* required is a comfortable pack that fits well and that is sturdy enough to carry the larger load and heavier weight required for an extended trip. Whether you use one of the older, tried-and-true external-frame packs or a newer internal-frame model is mostly a matter of personal preference. Volumes have been written on the advantages of one versus the other, but it really boils down to what you find most comfortable. Regardless of the type of pack you use, be sure to get a good rain cover to protect it against, well, the rain.

Clothing is covered in the section below, so the next most important item to discuss is a **backpacking tent.** Improvements in outdoors technology have probably done more for tents than for any other piece of equipment. Today you can purchase wonderful nylon creations that are remarkably sturdy, weigh only 3 or 4 pounds, and have plenty of sleeping room for two or more people. Decades ago people often tried to save weight by doing the trip with just a tarp. But you lose a lot of comfort that way and, with the new technology, you no longer save much weight. So forget the tarp and use a tent. Just make sure that the tent you use 1) has a good rain fly to protect you from the elements, 2) has a vestibule where you can place items such as your boots out of the rain, 3) has mosquito netting, and 4) has a waterproof floor. Most hikers also use a ground cloth to protect the tent floor from rocks and needles. If (and when) it rains, be sure to dry out your tent as soon as possible to prevent mold. Finally, if you are using a new tent, make sure to put it up in your backyard first, so you aren't forced to figure out how the darn poles work as a rainstorm is fast approaching, only to discover that you are two stakes short of being able to complete the job. (Don't ask me how I know this. Just take my word for it.)

A good **topographic map** is also a requirement. Do not rely on the free park brochure, which is designed for drivers and is wholly inadequate for backpackers. The old U.S. Geological

Survey topographic maps, though wonderfully detailed, are generally out of date and are not designed for hikers. Thus, the three best options for Wonderland Trail hikers are the Green Trails series maps (*Mount Rainier West #269* and *Mount Rainier East #270*), the Trails Illustrated map *Mount Rainier National Park,* and the Earthwalk Press *Hiking Map and Guide: Mt. Rainier National Park.* Of the three, the last is probably the best. All of these maps, which include mileages and highlight trails, camps, and other features useful for hikers, are available at local sporting goods stores, at bookstores in the park, or online from various outlets. Be sure to buy maps that are printed on waterproof and, preferably, tear-resistant paper or to carry the maps in a clear plastic covering.

As for **sleeping bags,** use one that is filled with synthetic material rather than down. Unfortunately, down bags, though wonderfully lightweight and warm, are useless if they get wet. Try to carry a bag that has a temperature rating of at least 32°F. If you are hiking in September, a bag with a rating of 20°F is a good investment. You should also consider bringing a lightweight liner to fit inside the bag. This will add an extra layer of warmth, make you more comfortable because your skin won't be up against a nylon surface, and help to keep the bag clean. Also, remember that wearing a wool knit cap while you sleep will make any sleeping bag feel much warmer.

About 50 feet of light **nylon cord** should be in every hiking party's supplies. You will need it to hang your food at some of the campsites along the way. It will also come in handy for improvised clotheslines, making repairs, and a variety of other uses.

For cooking, carry a small **backpacker's stove** as well as a pot and lightweight utensils. Remember when selecting the type of cookstove to use that you cannot mail or ship fuel in your food caches. Thus, you will probably have to carry all the cooking fuel for the entire trip from the start. Generally, white gas or butane stoves are the preferred choices. Also note that except in extreme emergencies, fires are prohibited in the backcountry of Mount Rainier National Park.

This might sound self-serving, but one other item you should strongly consider taking along is **this book.** It is designed, after all, to be compact and reasonably lightweight and holds a wealth of (hopefully) useful information that will make your trip more comfortable and enjoyable. To protect the book from the elements, cover it with clear self-adhesive paper (the stuff used to line shelves). If you are feeling generous to a certain guidebook author, you might also consider showing the book to other hikers and loudly extolling its virtues. But that's your call.

In the late 1980s outdoors equipment manufacturers had one of those "well, duh" epiphanies when they noticed that men and women are different. This belated discovery has dramatically improved life for female backpackers who were previously forced to use smaller versions of equipment designed for men. Today, women have a wide array of clothing, gear, and accessories that are specifically designed for their body shape and unique needs. So if it has been several years since those of you proudly sporting two X chromosomes have been backpacking, you might want to look into upgrading your equipment. The added comfort and utility of the new female-oriented gear may make the expense worthwhile.

Perhaps the two most important things to bring on your trip weigh nothing, but are often the hardest to obtain and the easiest to lose: common sense and the right attitude. More trips have been ruined by hikers getting injured after making poor choices or from unproductive grumbling about the rain or sore muscles than from any other cause. Simply avoiding dumb mistakes and having a positive attitude about the beauty of nature outweighing the inevitable discomforts of backpacking will make all the difference in the world.

CLOTHING

What you wear on your adventure will significantly affect your comfort on the trail, your ability to stay warm and dry, and even your survival should conditions get bad. There are all kinds of great hiking clothes on the market, but buying everything new would be prohibitively expensive. It is better to focus on just a few key items.

The first and most important article of clothing you will need for your trip around Mount Rainier is a high-quality pair of **hiking boots.** Although some people prefer to hike in running shoes on day hikes or short backpacking trips, these are not adequate for a long, tough trail such as the Wonderland. Your feet will get both wet and tired in running shoes, and the terrain will chew the shoes to pieces. So, even though they weigh more, you really should wear boots. There are many excellent brands that are made from either leather or tough waterproof and breathable synthetic materials, but anything that fits you comfortably and is waterproof will work well. It is usually wise to replace the factory insoles with a higher-quality product designed for rugged hiking.

The next wardrobe item is good **hiking socks.** Go with the thick wool-blend types that cushion your feet and wick moisture away to help prevent blisters. Many hikers like to wear two pairs for added comfort or to make their boots fit better. You should carry at least three or four pairs of socks and rinse them out regularly during your trip. An optional item to consider are gaiters, which protect your ankles and lower legs from water and brush and keep snow, mud, and small rocks from getting into your boots.

Now that you have taken care of the footwear, it's time to consider the rest of your body. Today's hiking clothes feature all kinds of terrific, high-tech fabrics that are lightweight, magically wick moisture away from your skin, resist getting smelly, and even, in some cases, have built-in insect repellent. In addition, even though the fabric is thin, the clothes are remarkably tough, protect you from the sun, are wind resistant, and dry very quickly. These are a huge improvement

Tiny creek below Mowich Lake

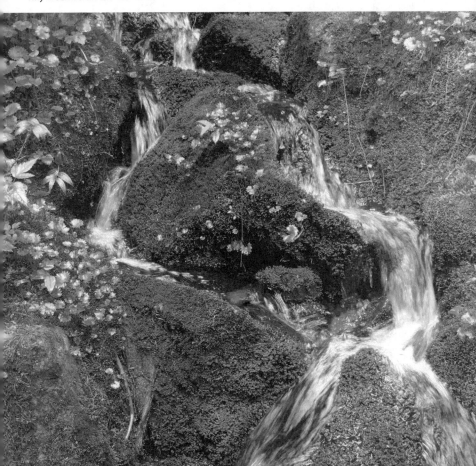

over the old cotton jeans and T-shirts, which once they got wet were worse than useless (often you were actually warmer going naked). By dressing in several lightweight layers it is relatively easy to remain comfortable in a variety of weather conditions and temperatures.

The **first layer** against your skin should be some kind of polypropylene, CoolMax, Capilene, or other synthetic material. These shirts are remarkably comfortable, retain heat even when they get wet, and wick away your perspiration on hot summer days. There are some excellent hiking shirts on the market that you can often wear separately without the need for a second outer layer. You must also carry, however, a long-sleeve hiking shirt to protect your skin from the sun and mosquitoes.

Perhaps even more important than your shirt is a good **rain jacket/Windbreaker.** This should be made from tough material that resists the rain yet allows your body to "breathe" so you won't be bathed in your own sweat. A variety of excellent materials are on the market to accomplish this trick. If you are going to be spending money on new clothes, make a good rain jacket a top priority, only after high-quality hiking boots and comfortable socks.

The final layer above the waist should be a **warm jacket.** Fleece is a good choice because it provides insulation with minimal weight. It can also be bundled up for use as a pillow. If you are hiking in late August or September, a second insulation layer, perhaps a wool sweater, would be a good idea. You should also bring a **hat** to protect from the sun and, as previously mentioned, a warm **wool knit cap.**

Below the waist, go with a pair of **hiking pants** that are made of the same tough wonder materials that dry quickly and resist the wind. Look for a pair that has plenty of pockets for snacks and other supplies and, if you like to hike in shorts, will convert into shorts by simply zipping off the lower legs. You might also want to bring a separate pair of **lightweight shorts or swim trunks** so you will have something to wear when you rinse out your hiking pants and hang them to dry. It is strongly advised that you also carry **rain pants,** which will protect your legs from water (both the rain and the heavy dew that often forms on plants in the morning) and provide a layer of warmth for your legs on cold evenings.

Some other optional clothing items to consider include a **bandanna, gloves or mittens** (especially late in the hiking season), and **lightweight camp shoes or sandals.** The last item adds tremendously to your comfort because, believe me, after a long day on the trail, it is close to heaven to slip out of your heavy hiking boots and into something lightweight and comfortable. They are also good for wearing when you cross streams, protecting your feet while still allowing you to keep your boots dry.

FOOD

The type of food you carry is based largely on your individual tastes. Wonderland Trail backpackers have successfully carried nothing but GORP (a mix of nuts, raisins, chocolate chips, and other items) for the entire trip while others prefer an array of fancy (and spendy) freeze-dried meals of everything from beef lasagna to pasta primavera. In general, take what tastes good to you, provides the necessary energy and nutrition, and is lightweight. Popular backpacking foods include instant rice or potato mixes, dried fruits and vegetables, jerky, granola and granola bars, energy bars, hard candies, instant soups and noodles, and various freeze-dried meals. Notice that fresh foods (apart from seasonal berries picked along the way) are not on the typical backpacker's menu. Unfortunately they are bulky and weigh far too much to be practical. In addition, fresh foods won't last more than a couple of days without refrigeration. As a result, it helps to bring along a few multivitamins to supplement your diet now that fresh fruits and vegetables have been removed.

Even though it adds to your pack's weight, take more food than you think you'll need. Backpacking uses lots of calories (among other things, the Wonderland Trail is one of the world's most scenic weight-loss programs), and you will need to replace those calories as you hike. Depending on your metabolism, your gender, and the difficulty of the terrain, as well as how cold the weather is and how far you hike each day, you will have to consume between 4,000 and 5,500 calories every day just to stay even. If (and when) it gets rainy and cold, you will have to eat additional food just to stay warm. Except for a few snacks at the Longmire store and possibly burgers at Sunrise Lodge, you will not be able to buy any food along the way. What you carry or send ahead in food caches is all you will have, so pack plenty.

It is also very important that you drink plenty of water. You should drink a minimum of 2 quarts of water per day and much more on hot days when hiking uphill. Remember that your body's thirst mechanism is not an adequate guide, so you should drink even if you do not feel thirsty. People tend to drink more when water is readily available, so many hikers use packs with hydration systems that have a water pouch inside and a tube that leads out to their mouth. Another good idea is to flavor your water with drink mixes. This will make it taste more interesting and help to replace some of the salts and other minerals that you sweat away as you hike.

CHECKLISTS

Required Items:

- [ ] permit
- [ ] backpack
- [ ] rain cover for pack
- [ ] sleeping bag
- [ ] sleeping pad or air mattress
- [ ] tent (with rain fly and mosquito netting)
- [ ] 1-quart water bottle (or hydration pouch)
- [ ] water filter or other water purifier
- [ ] money (for emergency phone calls and snacks)
- [ ] pocketknife
- [ ] sunscreen (SPF 15 or higher)
- [ ] insect repellent (not needed in late August or September)
- [ ] small flashlight/headlamp (with extra battery)
- [ ] 50 feet of nylon cord
- [ ] plastic signaling whistle
- [ ] small superabsorbent backpacker's towel
- [ ] waterproof stuff sacks/bear bags
- [ ] candle or other fire starter
- [ ] matches in a waterproof container
- [ ] stove, fuel, and cooking pot and utensils
- [ ] repair items (such as duct tape, needle and thread, and superglue)
- [ ] personal items (toothbrush and paste, medications and vitamins, lip balm—preferably with sun protection, toilet paper, dental floss, and so on)
- [ ] sunglasses/glacier glasses
- [ ] wallet
- [ ] car keys
- [ ] first-aid kit (including athletic tape, elastic bandage, bandages, antibiotic ointment, ibuprofen, Moleskin, antihistamine, safety pins, latex gloves, sterile gauze pads, and anti-diarrhea medicine)
- [ ] hiking boots (waterproof and with good insoles)
- [ ] socks (at least three to four pairs)
- [ ] long hiking pants (made from wind-resistant and fast-drying material)
- [ ] hiking shirt (long-sleeve)
- [ ] undershirt (made from wicking material—rinse daily)
- [ ] underwear (two pair, preferably of polypropylene)
- [ ] wool knit cap
- [ ] rain jacket/Windbreaker
- [ ] hat (for sun protection)
- [ ] food (your preferences, but bring plenty)
- [ ] topographic map
- [ ] compass
- [ ] common sense and the right attitude

Optional Items:

- [ ] this book
- [ ] camera (with extra battery and memory cards)
- [ ] cards, book to read, or other entertainment
- [ ] pen and paper

Optional Items (cont'd):

☐ small binoculars or monocular

☐ ground cloth for tent

☐ sleeping bag liner

☐ head net

☐ gaiters

☐ rain pants

☐ gloves/mittens

☐ wool sweater or vest (especially in September)

☐ bandanna

☐ lightweight camp shoes or sandals

☐ second hiking shirt or T-shirt

☐ second pair of hiking pants or shorts

☐ watch

☐ prescription glasses

☐ collapsible water container for around camp

☐ emergency space blanket (to bring on day hikes)

☐ wildflower or other nature guides

☐ walking stick(s)

☐ odorless hand lotion (for dry and cracking skin)

☐ small day pack for side trips (the top of many backpacks can be removed and used as a day pack)

☐ 1 or 2 large plastic garbage bags

Items to Leave Behind:

☐ fishing gear (there aren't many to catch)

☐ shaving items (no one cares if you look like Grizzly Adams)

☐ makeup and mirror (the former won't help much and the latter, well, you probably don't want to know)

☐ ice ax (unless you are traveling in early summer)

☐ cell phone and other electronic paraphernalia

☐ bear canister (usually too small to carry all of your food, and the bear poles and wires at the camps are sufficient)

☐ swimsuit (except perhaps in mid-August, the water is too cold for comfortable swimming)

☐ gun (technically legal to carry in the park but utterly useless)

☐ beer/alcohol

So how much will all of this weigh, or to put it another way, will your shoulders and hips ever forgive you? Personally, I never weigh my pack at the start of a long trip because I don't want to psych myself out by knowing how much weight I will be carrying. Those of you with less fragile psyches, however, may be interested to know that the total weight carried by a solo hiker, excluding food but including your pack, boots and clothing, a full quart of water, and all the cooking fuel you will need for the entire trip should come to between 30 and 35 pounds. Ten days of food will weigh something like 15 pounds, so if you start with all your food, then your pack will weigh just shy of an uncomfortable 50 pounds as you set out from the trailhead. Sending food caches ahead (see details on page 76) will reduce your starting weight accordingly. Also, you can reduce your load by sharing the weight of community items (water filter, nylon cord, cookstove and fuel, tent, first-aid kit, and the like) with a hiking partner.

How to Get to Mount Rainier

Compared with some of the more remote national parks in the United States, Mount Rainier is remarkably easy to reach. The park is located less than 100 miles from Seattle and all the amenities of civilization. Because of this proximity, the mountain is extremely popular as a day-trip destination for the more than 3 million residents of the Seattle area, which explains the huge crowds on summer weekends. See the locator map on page vi.

Despite the popularity, there is no public transportation to most trailheads in Mount Rainier National Park. To get here you must either drive your own vehicle or arrive on one of the many tour buses that visit the area from spring through fall. Unfortunately, those tour buses have a policy that they must return each day with the same number of people they started with, so hikers cannot use the service to be dropped off at the start of their trip. Therefore, for hikers who are flying in from out of town, the only realistic option for getting to the park is to rent a car.

There are several ways to access the park from Seattle, but the quickest way to reach Longmire from Seattle-Tacoma International Airport is to leave the airport and get onto

I-5 southbound. Drive 25 miles to the south end of Tacoma and take Exit 127 onto Washington Highway 512. Go east 2 miles, and then exit onto Washington Highway 7 and drive south for 35 miles to a junction just beyond the small town of Elbe. Go straight on Washington Highway 706 and proceed 14 miles, passing through Ashford, to the entrance station for Mount Rainier National Park. Continue east another 7 miles and then turn right into the Longmire complex. You will almost immediately pass a small sign for the Wonderland Trail, which goes to the left. The wilderness information center is another 75 yards away in a log building on the left. Lots of parking is nearby.

It is somewhat longer but still a reasonable drive if you are coming from Portland, Oregon. In this case, drive about 75 miles north on I-5 to Exit 68, where you turn onto US Highway 12. Drive 30 miles east to the town of Morton, and then go north on WA 7 for 17 miles to the junction beside the

Ptarmigan Ridge over Moraine Park

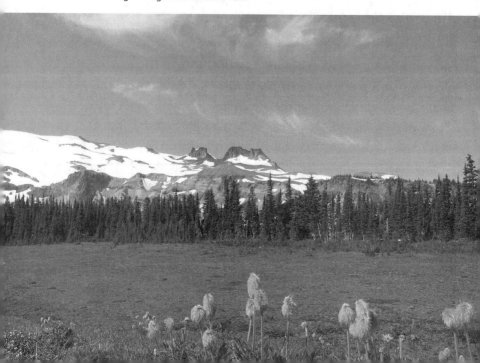

small town of Elbe. Turn right onto WA 706 and follow the directions to Longmire given beginning on page 71.

Hikers starting at Mowich Lake will find that it is a little trickier to locate. There are several possible approach routes, but probably the least confusing from the Seattle area is to go south on I-5 through Tacoma to Exit 127, where you turn east onto WA 512. Proceed 13 miles to a complicated intersection where you first go north on Washington Highway 167, and then almost immediately go right (east) onto Washington Highway 410, always following signs to Mount Rainier National Park. Drive 11 miles to a junction just before the town of Buckley, turn right onto Washington Highway 165, and proceed 2 miles to a junction with Washington Highway 162. Go left, staying on WA 165, and drive south for 8.9 miles, passing through the charming town of Wilkeson, to a possibly unsigned Y-junction. If you are heading to the Carbon River Ranger Station to pick up your wilderness permit, go left at the Y and proceed 8 miles to the park boundary and ranger station. To reach Mowich Lake, backtrack to the Y and take the right fork. The road remains paved for the next 1.7 miles and then turns to gravel and becomes bumpy and a little rough. The road proceeds uphill into the park and finally reaches the road-end parking lot at Mowich Lake, 17.1 miles from the Y.

If you are heading for Paradise, Sunrise, White River, Ohanapecosh, or any other destination in the park, simply follow the well-signed roads that are shown on both the maps in this book and on the free park brochure, which you receive upon entering the park.

Accommodations

Unless you arrive very early in the day, the odds are good that once you reach the park, you will need someplace to stay. Arriving in the afternoon and starting on the trail late in the day is possible but has two main problems associated with it. The first is that unless you called ahead, you are required to pick up your reserved permit by 10 a.m. on the day your trip is scheduled to begin or the permit is lost and the reserved campsites are given to other hikers on a first-come, first-serve basis. The second problem is that unless you start at Mowich Lake and spend the first night at Eagles Roost Camp (an easy 2-mile walk), you will have to cover at least 5 miles (and usually more) of mostly uphill terrain to reach the first allowable backpacker's campsite for the night. When burdened with the extremely heavy pack that is required at the start of your trip, this results in a particularly difficult first day. The best plan is to arrive in the area the day before, spend the night, and begin the next morning.

There are a variety of options for spending the night in or around Mount Rainier National Park. The park is home to two historic lodges: the National Park Inn at Longmire and the Paradise Inn at, where else, Paradise. The former is open year-round, but the Paradise Inn operates only during the summer months. These grand old facilities are very popular, so reservations are required, usually months in advance. For reservations at either lodge, contact Mount Rainier Guest Services ([360] 569-2275; **guestservices.com/rainier**). In Ashford, about 10 miles west of Longmire, there are several motels from which to choose. A few of the establishments are included in Appendix B, on page 183. Again, during the summer months, reservations are very helpful.

For those who want to camp, the park has four (possibly only three) car campgrounds: Cougar Rock, just a little up the road from Longmire; Ohanapecosh, in the southeast part of the park; and White River, in the northeast part of the park. Sunshine Point Campground, which was conveniently located just inside the park on the way to Longmire, was completely destroyed by floods in 2006. All that is left is a couple of forlorn-looking picnic tables stuck out on islands in the relocated river channel. The park is currently deciding if it will rebuild the campground at a new location or close it permanently. A small walk-in campground is located at Mowich Lake in the park's northwest corner. Several car campgrounds are on US Forest Service land outside of the park, but these are also very popular during the summer.

Car Shuttles

There are no commercial car-shuttle services on Mount Rainier. Of course, if you plan to do the entire Wonderland Trail, you will start and end at the same place so no car shuttle is required. Section hikers, however, will have to arrange transportation. Hitchhiking back to your starting point is neither feasible, advisable, nor, in some cases, legal. On the north and east sides of the mountain it is possible to do loops that combine the Wonderland Trail with the alternate routes for those sections, thus solving the car-shuttle dilemma because, once again, you start and end at the same location. See Chapter 4 for details on these hikes.

For the south and west sections of the Wonderland Trail, the only realistic option for section hikers is to arrange for a private car shuttle. The two most popular approaches are: 1) Have a friend drop you off at one end and pick you up at the other. This is most easily accomplished by people who live near the park and who can make the relatively short drive without undue time and expense. Frequently it is possible to find a friend who is heading to the mountain for a day hike and who will be happy to drop you off on his or her way. 2) Split up your party so that part of the group hikes in one direction and part in the other, with a planned meeting point in the middle to swap keys. You will need two permits for this approach because each party must have its own permit, but with some planning this can usually be accomplished. A variation on this option is to find someone whom you may not know but is a fellow hiker who, like you, is doing a section hike on the Wonderland Trail and similarly needs a way to get back where they started. The best ways to find such people are to post notices online with a local hiking club, such as The Mountaineers, or to put an ad in the club's newsletter.

Food Drops

A separate logistical issue to consider, and one for which your tired shoulders and hips will be very grateful, is caching food. You cannot expect to purchase food or other supplies along the way because the only locations where even basic supplies are available are at the Longmire general store and, seasonally, the lodge at Sunrise. Still, many hikers quite reasonably want to avoid beginning their journey with 10 or more days' worth of food and other supplies weighing down their progress. The obvious solution is to send your supplies ahead to locations where these food caches can be picked up along the way. Fortunately, this is reasonably easy to accomplish and, for hikers who follow the proper procedures, the National Park Service (NPS) is very good about helping with this task.

You can prepackage and send food caches by mail, UPS, or FedEx, or you can drop them off in person. In either case, you are required to pack your items in a hard-sided plastic container, which will keep rodents out of your food. Five-gallon buckets are a popular choice, though square Rubbermaid-type containers are also a possibility. Once you have picked up your supplies, the buckets are given to trail crews to assist in their work. **VERY IMPORTANT:** The container must be clearly labeled with your name, the number of your wilderness permit, the location at which the cache is to be picked up, and the date you will be retrieving it. When you eventually pick up the cached items, you will be required to sign for them. Any items that are not picked up are donated to local food banks at the end of the hiking season.

Fuel is considered a fire and safety hazard, so you are *not* allowed to mail or otherwise ship fuel as part of your food cache. If you want to store fuel for your stove, then you must deliver it in person. Most hikers simply carry all the fuel they need from the start.

The four locations along the Wonderland where food caches can be sent are the Longmire Wilderness Information Center, Mowich Lake Patrol Cabin, Sunrise Visitor Center, and White River Campground. Note that Sunrise and Mowich Lake generally do not open until early July. In addition, the Sunrise Visitor Center closes after Labor Day and the road into Mowich Lake can be closed because of snow as early as mid-September, so early and late-season hikers have fewer options.

Mail your food caches to the following addresses:
For the Longmire Wilderness Information Center:
Mount Rainier National Park
Longmire Wilderness Information Center
General Delivery
Longmire, WA 98397

For Mowich Lake (if you are using regular mail):
Mount Rainier National Park
Carbon River Ranger Station
P.O. Box 423
Wilkeson, WA 98396

For Mowich Lake (for UPS or FedEx deliveries):
Mount Rainier National Park
Carbon River Ranger Station
Fairfax Forest Reserve Road E
Carbonado, WA 98323

Rangers will deliver your food to the storage bin behind the Mowich Lake Patrol Cabin before your designated pickup date.

For either the Sunrise Visitor Center or White River Campground:
    Mount Rainier National Park
    White River Wilderness Information Center
    70002 Washington Highway 410 E
    Enumclaw, WA 98022

Based on the information shown on the outside of the container, rangers will deliver your food cache to the appropriate location before your planned pickup date. *Note:* For White River Campground the food storage bin is located behind the ranger station.

Getting in Shape and Pacing Yourself

If you are new to backpacking, then I must be blunt here: *Do not* think of the Wonderland Trail as a suitable choice for your first foray into the backcountry, no matter how enticing it may sound. Put simply, the trail ain't easy and requires way too much effort, experience, planning, potentially expensive gear, and difficult conditioning for first-timers to enjoy their trip, or even to attempt it safely. Plan to do several warm-up trips first to see if you really enjoy the sport and want to invest the time, sweat, and expense into tackling the Wonderland Trail. Another option, as discussed previously, is to break the trail into shorter and more manageable sections.

There are two issues when it comes to getting in shape for a trip around Mount Rainier. The first and more obvious one is physical conditioning. Unless you are already in backpacking shape, be prepared to do some work to get your legs, lungs, and other body parts strong enough to do the trail in reasonable comfort. As with any activity, the best way to get in shape for hiking and backpacking is to go hiking and backpacking. That probably sounds obvious, but you might be surprised how many people mistakenly try to prepare for backpacking by, say, swimming or lifting weights. Those are fine activities and will certainly help with the cardiovascular and strength demands of carrying a pack over rough terrain, but they're no substitute for the real thing. So get out on the trails. Do plenty of day hikes over gradually longer distances and carrying an increasingly heavy load. Then take some short backpacking trips to get the feel of the pack on your body. Once you can comfortably hike 7–10 miles a day, gaining at least 2,000 feet while carrying a heavy pack, then you should be able to handle the Wonderland Trail. With proper

Stafford Falls

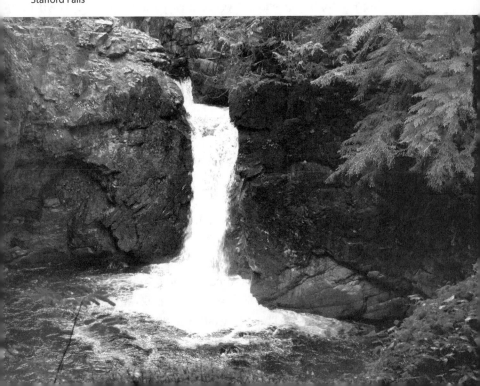

conditioning, completing the trail is within the physical abilities of just about anybody, from children as young as 11 or 12 to grandmothers in their 70s. It may require some work to get there, but the rewards are well worth it.

The second, less obvious (but no less important) issue when it comes to getting in shape for the Wonderland Trail is mental conditioning. You need to make sure your mind is prepared for day after day of relative solitude, for the constant company of only one or two companions (who will inevitably get on your nerves), for sleeping in the dark with thoughts of bears or bugs creeping around just outside the tent, and for convincing yourself that even though you are tired and it's cold and possibly raining outside, it is nonetheless time to get up and tackle the day. Even though issues like these are, admittedly, all in your head, that does not make them any less crucial to a successful and enjoyable trip than issues that are all in your feet, your knees, or anywhere else. There is no better way for you to test your ability to deal with these crucial mental skills than to go on several shorter backpacking trips before you take on the Wonderland Trail.

Once on the trail, an equally important issue is setting a comfortable and sustainable pace. Far too many people—a remarkably high percentage of whom are young males—set out like a racehorse and end up dragging along like a swaybacked nag long before they reach their destination. In general, a steady, moderate pace is your best bet for maximum enjoyment on the trail. Most reasonably fit hikers average around 2 miles per hour, which, when combined with rest stops and time to smell the flowers and enjoy the scenery, adds up to a very manageable 7-hour (or so) day to hike 10 miles, a good average distance for the spacing of your campsites. Keep in mind, however, that the Wonderland Trail is almost never flat. There is well over 22,000 feet of elevation gain and loss along the way, and all this up and down will dramatically affect your pace. I like to average a steady, plodding 1.5 miles per hour when going uphill and a more vigorous 2.5 miles per hour on downhills. If any given day involves a great deal of elevation gain or loss, then adjust your time estimates accordingly to figure out how long it will take you to reach camp. As previously mentioned, it is also crucial that you allow time for rest breaks. This is important not only to allow your body and mind to recover from the exertion, but also so you can appreciate the scenery, take plenty of pictures, enjoy the wildlife, and do all the other things that are, after all, why you came on the trip in the first place.

Permits

To protect from overuse, the NPS imposes a limited-use permit system on overnight backcountry travel. Day hikers do not need a permit, but because you cannot do the Wonderland Trail as a day hike (or even, realistically, as a series of very long day hikes), this doesn't help you. During the short two-month hiking season, the demand for overnight permits is quite high. As a result, obtaining a permit to hike when and where you want to go may be the most difficult hurdle you must overcome.

While 30% of all overnight wilderness permits are given out on a first-come, first-serve basis, the majority, approximately 70%, are reserved in advance. Thus, your best bet is to make a reservation.

The reservation process is straightforward and fairly simple. Starting on March 15 of each year, reservation requests are accepted by fax, letter, or in person at the Longmire Wilderness Information Center. No phone or e-mail reservations are accepted. Though the wilderness permit itself is free, there is a $20 per party fee for reservations (up to a maximum of 12 persons), which can be paid by check or with any major credit card. The reservation fee is nonrefundable, even if you end up being unable to make the trip. Reservations can be made for trips of up to 14 consecutive days. Starting on April 1, all reservation requests that the park has received between March 15 and April 1 are put into a bin and processed in random order. Therefore, there is no advantage to sending in your request on March 15 as opposed to, say, March 26. Any requests made after April 1 are processed in the order they are received. Because the park receives several hundred reservation requests during the initial period and has a limited number of rangers available to process them, it usually takes several weeks before all the reservations are finished and confirmation letters are sent out. So don't expect to hear anything until about May. The simplest way to obtain a blank reservation form is to print one off the park's website at **tinyurl.com/wonderlandres**. After completing the form, send it by fax to (360) 569-3131 or by mail to Mount Rainier National Park, Wilderness Information Center, 55210 238th Avenue E, Ashford, WA 98304-9751.

Given the number of reservation requests and the limited number of available campsites, not all requests can be fulfilled. Try to be as flexible as possible and be willing to accept different starting dates or different campsites than what you originally wanted. If the park is unable to fulfill your request, they will send you a letter to that effect and no reservation fee will be charged. Successful requesters receive a confirmation letter, but this is *not* your permit. When you arrive, you must stop at a ranger station or wilderness information center to pick up your actual permit. Any reserved permits that are not picked up by 10 a.m. on the day that the trip is scheduled to begin will be canceled and the available campsites given to other people on a first-come, first-serve basis. If you plan to arrive later than

10 a.m., you must call to let the park know in advance so you do not lose your permit. Finally, the park allows for one change to a confirmed reservation, but only if the changes to dates or campsites can be accommodated without displacing other confirmed reservations (often very difficult, so expect to be disappointed). There is no additional fee charged for the first change. Any further changes to your plans will incur an additional $20 reservation fee.

If you did not make a reservation, then your only option is to get a first-come, first-serve permit. Just like it sounds, this involves showing up at one of the wilderness information centers or ranger stations, getting in line, and hoping to snag one of the available spaces. You can get a permit for a trip starting either that day or up to one day before your planned starting date. Remember that even if you are the first in line, not all camps set aside for first-come, first-serve permits will necessarily be available. Frequently someone will have already taken the available campsite for a trip that started two or three days before your planned hike. **Tip:** If your trip is in mid-September or later, then obtaining a first-come, first-serve permit is a reasonable option because demand for permits has dropped considerably by then and you can usually get into the campsites you want. In July and August, however, this can be very difficult, so do not plan to fly across the country and simply show up at a ranger station assuming you can get a permit. It may turn out to be a wasted trip.

In the past, Wonderland Trail hikers who were unable to obtain a permit to camp in one of the designated campsites along the trail could get a permit to camp in one of the park's adjoining cross-country camping zones instead. This is no longer allowed for Wonderland Trail thru-hikers, so once the trailside camps are full, you are out of luck. In fact, even if you *prefer* to camp away from the trail in a cross-country zone, or feel that a particular camping zone will be more scenic or a better fit with your planned hiking schedule, the park will not allow this and will not give you a permit.

When obtaining a permit it is very important to remember that, barring an emergency, you are expected to adhere to your permit itinerary. If you are scheduled to camp at a particular place on a particular night, then that is where you must be. If that means hiking in a driving rainstorm all day to get there, then so be it. Taking an unscheduled layover day is not allowed because someone else almost certainly has a permit to camp in the place you were supposed to leave. Rangers are adamant that hikers stick with their permit schedule. If you think you will need a layover day along the way (a great idea, if you have the time), then include it in your original permit request.

Leave No Trace Principles and Backcountry Etiquette

Mount Rainier National Park is a public treasure that we all have a responsibility to protect and preserve. In general, responsible hikers have very little impact on the land, and it is important that we keep it that way, not only to protect this wonderful environment but also to ensure access for future generations. For decades the credo has been to "leave no trace" of your passage, but the time has come to go beyond these now-familiar principles and to actually leave the land in *better* shape than before we arrived. Here are some guidelines; many are required by park rules and all are required to be a good backcountry citizen.

- Do not bury or leave behind any kind of litter, even biodegradable items such as eggshells or orange peels. Even better, remove any litter left by others (blessedly little these days).

- Do some minor trail maintenance as you hike: kick rocks off the trail, remove limbs and debris, and drain water from the path to reduce mud and erosion. Report major trail-maintenance problems, such as large blowdowns or washouts, to the land managers so they can concentrate their limited dollars where they are most needed.

- Always camp in designated sites along the trail and place your tent either on the established tent pads or on compacted soils where others have camped before.

- Never feed wildlife (that includes birds and squirrels, no matter how cute they look or how much they beg) and encourage others to refrain.

- Never walk off-trail in meadows, especially at higher elevations, to avoid trampling the fragile plants and wildflowers.

- Never cut across any of the several hundred switchbacks you encounter along the Wonderland Trail.

- Travel in smaller groups and always be respectful of the desire of other hikers for solitude and quiet. (Don't talk loudly on the trail or late into the night around camp. Don't let your kids yell across a lake. Carry a tent that is a natural color. You get the idea.)

- Never use soap, even biodegradable soap, in or near *any* natural water source. Wash your body by simply splashing water over yourself, and wash dishes by carrying water well away from creeks or lakes and scrubbing them clean in a forested area.

- Do not build campfires. They are prohibited by park rules and are damaging to the land.

- Finally, forget any outdated attitudes you may have about going out to "conquer" the wilderness. This isn't a war and the land cannot survive very many "conquerors."

Other Items Worth Considering

Those of you who like to hike with your dog should be aware that pets are not allowed on the Wonderland or any other backcountry trail in Mount Rainier National Park. Sorry, Fido, you'll have to sit this one out.

To protect the environment, fires are not allowed anywhere in the backcountry of Mount Rainier National Park. For cooking use a small backpacker's stove, and for warmth bring along an extra sweater or take a brisk walk in the evening to get the blood flowing.

Sadly, in my view, today's pervasive technology seems to have given people the impression that they simply *must* be calling, texting, tweeting, or whatever with family, friends, coworkers, and seemingly every other person on the planet 24/7. Increasingly, this attitude even applies when people are in the backcountry. Sorry, folks, but it's time for an attitude adjustment. Cell phone coverage along the Wonderland Trail is described by rangers as "spotty at best," and, shockingly enough, none of the campsites offer Wi-Fi. I know this may be hard to believe for some of you, but you simply won't be able to call, get on the Internet, chat with Facebook friends, or do most anything else technology-related for the duration of your trip. Most rational people just leave the electronics at home, seeing little reason to carry around what effectively acts as a paperweight. You might even find the technology-free interlude to be a good experience. Remember, one reason people go to the backcountry is for a break from the rat race. So leave the electronic "rats" at home and enjoy the wonders of the natural world instead.

People sometimes ask about bringing a GPS device on the trail. Until at least mid-July there are usually some places along the Wonderland Trail where large snowfields can make navigation challenging and a GPS might come in handy. For most of the hiking season, however, the Wonderland Trail is both well maintained and well signed, so few hikers have any difficulty keeping on the proper course. Once in a while you may temporarily encounter difficult weather conditions such as thick fog or, very rarely, whiteout conditions in a snowstorm where you might need some help in keeping on course. In the summer such weather is unusual, however, and is almost always temporary, so for the most part you can simply make a quick shelter and wait it out. Thus, there is usually no need to carry the extra weight of a GPS. A small compass, and the skills to use it, should be adequate for most hikers.

The standard advice in guidebooks is that you should never hike alone. It is generally assumed that this recommendation is for safety reasons, but while there is some safety in numbers, the main reason not to go backpacking alone is mental. Human beings are social animals. Most people enjoy backpacking (or any activity) much more if they have along at least one compatible companion with whom they can share the day's experiences. Having a hiking partner will also make your journey more comfortable because you can lighten your load by sharing the weight of community items. That said, hundreds of experienced solo backpackers (including me) have safely completed the Wonderland Trail, so if you lack the sales skills to talk friends or family into coming along, that does not necessarily mean you shouldn't make the trip. You will meet many interesting folks both along the trail and at camp in the evening with whom you can swap stories and gain that necessary human companionship. For safety reasons, however, if you have only limited experience on the trail, the never-hike-alone advice should be taken to heart.

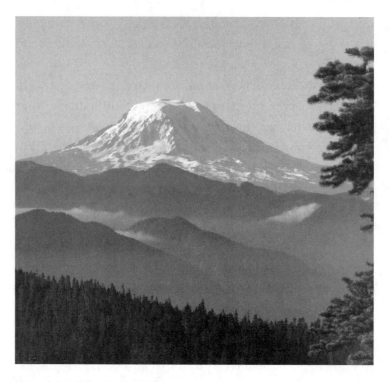

Mount Adams from Cowlitz Divide

Out-of-staters who are flying into Seattle to do the Wonderland Trail will have to purchase cooking fuel after they arrive. It is dangerous and illegal to carry or ship fuel on airplanes. There are numerous excellent sporting goods stores in the Seattle-Tacoma area that sell fuel for any type of stove. (See Appendix B, on page 183, for addresses and directions.) Do not wait until you get in or near the park to buy fuel, as the few stores that carry it may be out, and it will be much more expensive than it is in the city. Also remember to carry items that the Transportation Safety Administration considers potential weapons (such as a pocketknife) in your checked baggage rather than with your carry-on items, so these are not confiscated at the airport.

AVOID TUNNEL VISION: TAKE THE SIDE TRIPS

To make sure that you have the best possible trip, I feel obliged to provide one final piece of invaluable advice from someone who has hiked the Wonderland Trail many times: don't be a slave to the official tread. It is certainly true that even hikers who never leave the official Wonderland Trail will enjoy a terrific trip with great scenery and memories to last a lifetime. Your hike will be tremendously enhanced, however, if you include as many side trips as your time and schedule allow. Much of the park's best scenery is a short distance *off* the Wonderland Trail on side trails and unofficial boot paths that lead to generally uncrowded glory spots with spectacular views, lots of wildlife, and tremendous photo opportunities.

To hike the trail without making the side trips to Mirror Lakes, the viewpoint above Sunset Park, and the ridge below Willis Wall, for example, would be a real shame. Throughout Chapter 4, I have highlighted what in my experience are the best and most rewarding shorter side trips in special Side Trip Alert boxes. Though dozens of other excellent side trips are possible, if you include as many of these highlighted adventures as you can, your hike will be infinitely more enjoyable and rewarding.

When taking compass readings in Mount Rainier National Park, be sure to take into account the local magnetic declination of approximately 16.5 degrees east (as of 2010). This has been changing at a rate of about 0 degrees and 9 minutes west every year for the last few decades due to a slow shift in the location of the magnetic North Pole.

Finally, on any trip of this length your last-minute checklist is likely to be long: lots of packing and weighing, letting a responsible person know of your plans and when you expect to return, stopping your mail delivery, and dozens of other items. While I do not wish to add to your chores, I will point out something that far too many hikers forget to do just before a long trip: trim your toenails. It will save your feet lots of discomfort and, believe me, you will find that performing this chore on the trail with nothing but a pocketknife is extremely difficult.

Opposite: Mount Rainier from lower Spray Park

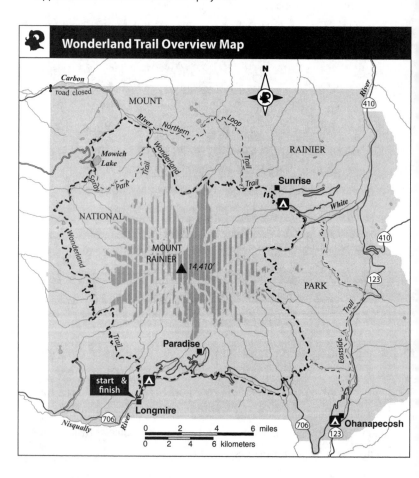

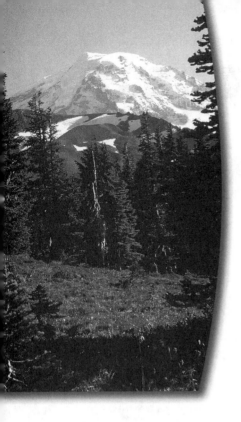

𝄞 *4* 𝄞
Trail Description

Note: Mileages exclude detours to photo spots, spur trails to campsites, and any of the many possible side trips. As previously mentioned, the mileages also change every year due to detours around washouts and the varying placement of seasonal bridges. Therefore, think of these mileages as only general guides, recognizing that the actual distance you hike will almost certainly be greater.

Section 1
Longmire to Mowich Lake
DISTANCE...34.1 miles

A majority of those who hike the entire Wonderland Trail begin at Longmire and travel clockwise. Thus, the first section you will probably tackle is around the west side of the mountain between Longmire and Mowich Lake. This is a

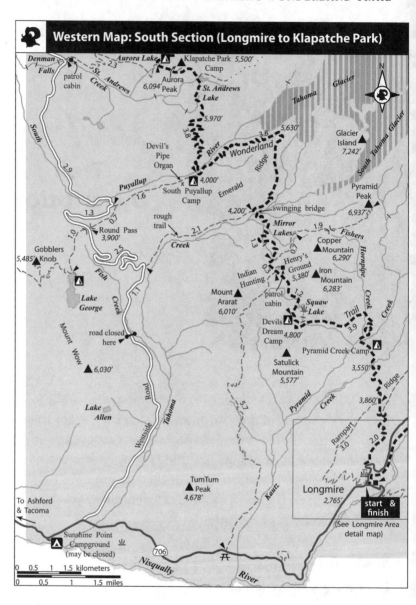

Western Map: South Section (Longmire to Klapatche Park)

long and relatively tough section, with lots of ups and downs and some steep trails. It is also outstandingly beautiful, so you don't have to wait to get to the good stuff. The scenery at Indian Henry's Hunting Ground, Emerald Ridge, Klapatche Park, and Sunset Park is as good or better than anything else in the park, or just about anywhere else in the United States for that matter. Surprisingly, this section also provides solitude. With the permanent closure of the flood-prone Westside Road, day hikers can no longer reasonably explore most of the trails here. As a result, Wonderland Trail hikers typically share the scenery only with other backpackers.

Before setting out, it's worth investing a little time checking out the historic buildings around Longmire, formerly the park's headquarters. The two most important of the many log structures here, at least for the hiker, are the Longmire Museum and the Longmire Wilderness Information Center, both about 75 yards from the Wonderland Trailhead. The small museum offers fascinating displays on the natural and human history of Mount Rainier National Park and includes a gift shop where you can pick up postcards, a wildflower guide, or that ever-popular T-shirt. The museum is directly across the Longmire access road from the Wonderland Trailhead and is open 9 a.m.–5 p.m. daily July 1– September 5 and 9 a.m.–4:30 p.m. the rest of the year. The wilderness information center is just east of the trailhead and is where you should go to pick up your reserved permit (or ask about a first-come, first-serve permit) and to inquire about the latest trail and weather conditions. The facility is open 7:30 a.m.–5 p.m. daily July 1–October 10.

The Wonderland Trail starts beside a small sign just a few yards east of where the Longmire access road leaves the Longmire-Paradise Road (also known as Washington Highway 706). Ascending gradually through a typical low-elevation forest dominated by western hemlocks, Douglas firs, and western red cedars, the wide trail climbs beside the road for 0.1 mile before splitting to start the loop.

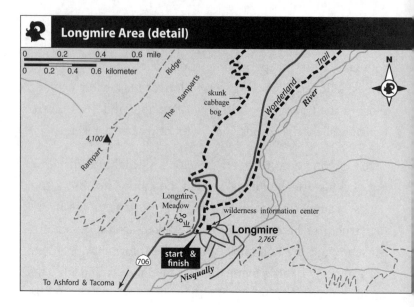

For the clockwise loop you bear left at the fork and continue paralleling the road for just less than 0.2 mile to a crossing of the highway, where the road makes a sharp right turn beside a small upper parking lot. Here you leave the road, and your wilderness adventure begins.

The route starts with an uphill that, initially at least, is quite gentle beneath a shady canopy of large evergreens. The undergrowth is an interesting mix of, among other species, deer ferns, various mosses, foamflowers, blueberries, and one small bog of skunk cabbage. The last plant graces the forest with huge, shiny, dark-green leaves and prefers wet areas at relatively low elevations. In early summer this plant has large, showy, yellow flowers. Though the odor from these blossoms is not nearly as offensive as that from the plant's namesake, it is also unlikely to be the basis for a perfume any time soon. As with many perennially wet places along the trail, you cross the bog on a log puncheon bridge.

In several places the trail passes large, old conifers that have fallen prey to time and winds, dropping to the forest floor and exposing massive root systems that are interesting (and a bit humbling) to examine. As is typical in old-growth forests, the downed trees often become nurse logs, providing their stored nutrients to a new generation of trees.

After the skunk cabbage bog the trail becomes noticeably steeper as you make your way toward the top of Rampart Ridge. The ascent (only the first of many, so get used to it) includes seven switchbacks to help lessen the steepness. These zigzags in the trail are another feature you must get used to, as there are hundreds more to negotiate over the next 91 or so miles. A little before the top of this first 1,100-foot climb is a junction with Van Trump Park Trail, which branches to the right.

You go straight, still gaining elevation, and after 0.2 mile reach a junction at the top of the ridge. The Rampart Ridge Trail angles in from the left. You go straight and for the next 0.4 mile gain or lose very little elevation on the gentle, woodsy route before descending five well-graded switchbacks to relatively clear Kautz Creek. As will be true for dozens of creeks and rivers along the Wonderland Trail, spring floods cause the stream to regularly change course, shifting its channel to different places in its wide, boulder-strewn riverbed. To accommodate, trail crews annually reroute the path around washouts and install a seasonal log bridge over the channel chosen by the creek in any given year. Without an established tread it can be a challenge for hikers to locate the proper course amid the rocks, so watch for cairns (little piles of rocks used to mark the route) and look on the other side of the riverbed for the renewal of the trail. On the plus side, the opening in the forest offers your first full-on view of Mount Rainier rising majestically to the north-northeast.

Once back in forest, and on unambiguous trail, you gradually gain elevation for 0.2 mile and then come to the signed turn-off for the recently relocated Pyramid Creek Camp on your right. This is the first of dozens of designated campsites along the trail, and Wonderland Trail thru-hikers are required to camp in these locations during their trip. Like the others, Pyramid Creek Camp is a comfortable place with numbered sites for camping and a bear pole to hang your food. Most (but not quite all) campsites also have a toilet, a good nearby source of water, and established tent pads.

The Wonderland Trail goes straight at the junction with the Pyramid Creek Camp turnoff and wanders along for another 0.2 mile before coming to the log bridge over Pyramid Creek. The slightly silty creek is the first of many you'll encounter that resembles the color of chocolate milk. The color is the result of all the silt and glacial flour the stream is carrying away from glaciers upstream.

Shortly after the bridge over Pyramid Creek you cross Fishers Hornpipe Creek, a clearer stream that, like other nonglacial streams, is a superior source of water to silt-laden Pyramid Creek. Now you begin the trip's next big uphill, which gains almost 1,900 feet over the next 3.3 miles. First up are 11 fairly steep switchbacks that take you to a bridged crossing of clear and babbling Fishers Hornpipe Creek. From here an extended uphill traverse takes you to a bridge over small Devils Dream Creek, and then a short set of switchbacks leads to an unseen waterfall on your right that drops into a deep and narrow chasm. A few more steep, rounded turns lead you past another unnamed falls to the lower end of Devils Dream Camp, a large area of several sites spread out on the hillside over the next 0.15 mile. The camp is the traditional first night for Wonderland Trail hikers. **Tip:** If you still

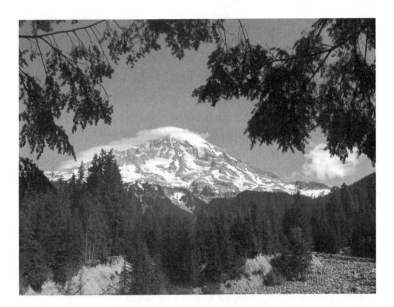

Mount Rainier from Kautz Creek

have some energy, set up your tent, grab your camera, and then continue hiking 1.2 miles to Indian Henry's Hunting Ground on the afternoon of your first day. Photographs across the glorious meadow up to the mountain are usually better with the afternoon sun *behind* you rather than in the blinding morning light the next day.

About 0.4 mile past Devils Dream Camp the forest opens up as you pass the wet meadows and shallow ponds of the Squaw Lakes. The craggy butte that rises to the northeast above these lakes is Iron Mountain. Another 0.7 mile of uphill takes you to Indian Henry's Hunting Ground, the first of countless classic beauty spots you will visit on the mountain. This one is a rolling meadowland with millions of wildflowers, a few small ponds, and many scattered trees. There is a superb view across the meadows to the rugged double summit of Mount Rainier. It's a view that is well worth a long rest stop to fully appreciate. About 0.1 mile into your hike across this paradise is a junction with Kautz Creek Trail, which goes left.

You go straight and 100 yards later reach the short side trail that goes right to the Indian Henry's Ranger Station/Patrol Cabin. A wilderness ranger is usually stationed here for most of the summer. Sticking with the Wonderland Trail, you come to a junction with Mirror Lakes Trail just 0.3 mile after the turnoff to the patrol cabin.

SIDE TRIP ALERT:
MIRROR LAKES AND PYRAMID PEAK

Turning right at this junction takes you on a 0.7-mile one-way side trip through meadows to the Mirror Lakes. Though little more than small ponds, these four pools offer wonderful views across their waters to Mount Rainier. It is, in fact, one of the most historically important and well-known views in the park because this was the spot chosen by the artist Asahel Curtis to depict the mountain in a postage stamp commemorating the park in 1934. The view is just as spectacular today as it was when Curtis photographed his famous scene. If you are feeling up for a tough but highly rewarding climb, consider continuing your side trip beyond the Mirror Lakes. Though the official trail ends at the lakes, an obvious and easy-to-follow path continues beyond, gaining very little elevation for the next 0.6 mile as it goes around the northeast side of Copper Mountain. After crossing a grassy saddle, the trail makes a steep, switchbacking climb that ascends 1,350 feet in the next 1.3 miles to a stunning viewpoint atop 6,937-foot Pyramid Peak. The up-close and personal look at the dramatic southwest face of Mount Rainier and its flowing mantle of glaciers is positively overwhelming.

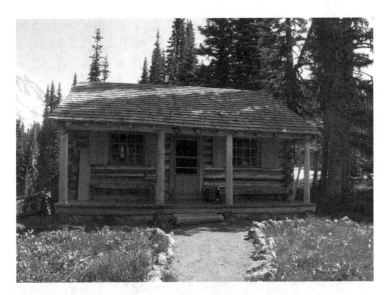

Indian Henry's Patrol Cabin

Back on the Wonderland Trail, you go north from the Mirror Lakes junction, soon leave the wonderful meadows of Indian Henry's Hunting Ground, and begin a sometimes-steep descent. It starts with three short switchbacks, then a traverse where you cross a small creek in the middle of a segmented waterfall. After nine more switchbacks you cross a log over a clear little creek. **Tip:** Be sure to fill your water bottles, as this is the last reliable clear water for the next few miles, including a tough climb over Emerald Ridge.

Below the creek crossing you go down 10 more short switchbacks to the colossal swinging bridge across rampaging Tahoma Creek. The 250-foot-long bridge, with its tall metal towers and cable-suspended (and very narrow) wooden plank surface is an engineering marvel, though it might not seem that way as you struggle with motion sickness and vertigo when you cross the seemingly unstable span. This is the longest, possibly the scariest, and certainly the most memorable bridge on the Wonderland Trail. For safety, cross one at a time, so you don't cause dangerous bouncing or swaying in the bridge for other hikers. **Tip:** It's a good idea to stow away your walking stick(s), so you have both hands free to hold on to the thin wire railings while you cross.

After regaining your land legs on the north side of Tahoma Creek, you soon reach a junction with Tahoma Creek Trail. The once-popular path has been washed out so frequently that the National Park Service (NPS) no longer maintains the trail. Today, the route is quite rough and has lots of ups and downs, but it remains passable for careful and experienced hikers.

Swinging bridge over Tahoma Creek

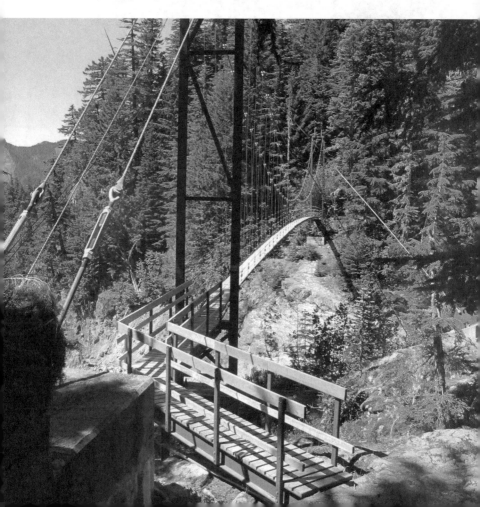

You go right at the Tahoma Creek junction and begin the next long uphill. Much of the climb is rocky and exposed to the sun, so it can be hot on summer afternoons. There are four widely spaced switchbacks over the first 0.8 mile where the trail is still partly shaded by trees. Once you get above the trees, however, the landscape is all rocks, snowfields, and meadows ending with three switchbacks just below the top. All the sweat is worth it, though, once you top out on Emerald Ridge with its dramatic up-close look at Mount Rainier and great views down onto the ice of Tahoma Glacier in the canyon to the north. Much of the glacier is covered with yellow and orange rocks, which add more color to the countless wildflowers on the ridge itself. To the southeast rise the high cliffs of Glacier Island, so named because until recent decades of glacial retreat, the Tahoma and South Tahoma Glaciers went all the way around the butte and met at its base, making it an island of rock surrounded by ice. To the northeast a tall waterfall drops onto the rocks and ice on the other side of Tahoma Glacier. If you can tear your eyes away from the smashing scenery (good luck!), Emerald Ridge is a good place to look for mountain goats.

The trail now descends, very steeply at times, down the northwest side of Emerald Ridge. **Warning:** The tread here is often covered with loose gravel, which makes for treacherous footing, so take small steps and be very cautious on the descent. I once met a battered hiker who nicknamed this downhill section "the roller derby" because she felt as though she was on skates the whole time, and after two bad falls, she had the bruises of a typical roller derby participant.

In the exposed and treeless upper part of the descent, there are a dozen tight little switchbacks. After that, you reenter forest and make numerous twists, turns, and switchbacks as you continue rapidly losing elevation. Just before the bottom of the long descent, and 2.2 miles from the top, you reach a junction with South Puyallup Trail. To reach South Puyallup Camp, walk 50 yards down the trail to the left.

SIDE TRIP ALERT: DEVIL'S PIPE ORGAN

Even if you are not staying at South Puyallup Camp, it is well worth taking the South Puyallup Trail and walking about 0.1 mile past the camp to view an extremely impressive display of columnar andesite (a type of volcanic rock) that rises in tall cliffs on the left (south) side of the trail. The area has no official name but is sometimes referred to as the Devil's Pipe Organ.

Back on the Wonderland Trail, the path soon takes you down to a sturdy wooden bridge over the South Puyallup River, a glacial stream that resembles a thick milk shake with a yellowish-brown color. The trail then ascends the next ridge on eight long and generally well-graded switchbacks, most of the way either in forest or across brushy slopes. At the top of the ridge the trail makes another sharp right-turning switchback and then follows the ascending ridgetop into increasingly open and interesting terrain on a course directly toward Mount Rainier. After about 0.4 mile the trail veers left, leaving the ridge, and descends two lazy switchbacks. You cross a small snowmelt creek, and then spend the next 0.3 mile regaining some of your recently lost elevation across open slopes that provide excellent views to the west of the Puget Sound area. At the top of the short uphill is St. Andrews Lake. The small lake offers views across its waters to Mount Rainier, but the water often remains covered with ice well into August. Immediately north of St. Andrews Lake is a sign that says simply WONDERLAND TRAIL with arrows pointing both right and left.

SIDE TRIP ALERT: ST. ANDREWS PARK

Right behind the WONDERLAND TRAIL sign is an unmaintained but obvious boot path that goes east across the meadow-covered hillside north of St. Andrews Lake. The circuitous route climbs about 0.6 mile into the high basin east of St. Andrews Lake. Here you are treated to several small ponds, lovely meadows, and outstanding views. The route also provides access to steep but fun off-trail wandering in the alpine terrain around Tokaloo Spire, Tokaloo Rock, and the ridge between Tahoma and Puyallup Glaciers.

From St. Andrews Lake the Wonderland Trail travels north about 0.2 mile before coming to a cliff-top viewpoint with an outstanding view of Mount Rainier and down into the yawning depths of the canyon of North Puyallup River. The trail then descends gently for almost another mile before reaching a saddle overlooking Aurora Lake. Here, there is another sign reading WONDERLAND TRAIL with arrows pointing left and right.

SIDE TRIP ALERT: AURORA PEAK

Immediately behind the WONDERLAND TRAIL sign is another boot path, this time going uphill to the northeast. The very steep route ascends the mostly open and rocky slopes of Aurora Peak, gaining 450 feet in less than 0.4 mile to the summit. This is a superb side trip, especially late in the day, because at the top you have a dramatic up-close look at the entire craggy and glacier-covered west face of Mount Rainier. It is a wonderful spot to sit and admire the drama of this great mountain.

From the little saddle beside Aurora Peak the Wonderland Trail descends an open slope for a little more than 0.1 mile to a junction with St. Andrews Creek Trail beside the outlet of gorgeous Aurora Lake. The small lake sits in the middle of a flat meadow called Klapatche Park and provides a view across its waters to spire-shaped Tokaloo Rock and ice-covered Mount Rainier. The Wonderland Trail goes to the right.

Late in the evening Klapatche Park is one of the best places on the mountain to enjoy the alpenglow as the light of sunset turns the mountain pink. To fully appreciate the show, of course, you have to spend the night here and, fortunately, you can do just that at nearby Klapatche Park Camp. To find the camp, go north on the Wonderland Trail from the St. Andrews Creek junction and walk 100 feet along the northwest side of Aurora Lake. The small camp is popular, so you may have a hard time getting a permit to stay here, but it's worth trying.

Mount Rainier and Aurora Lake

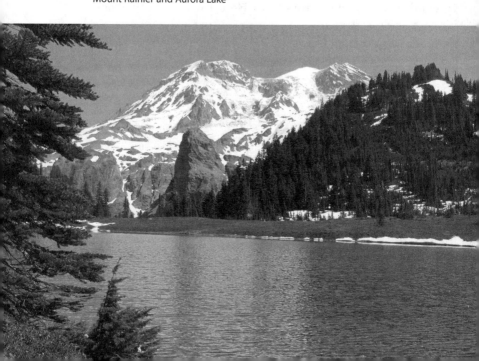

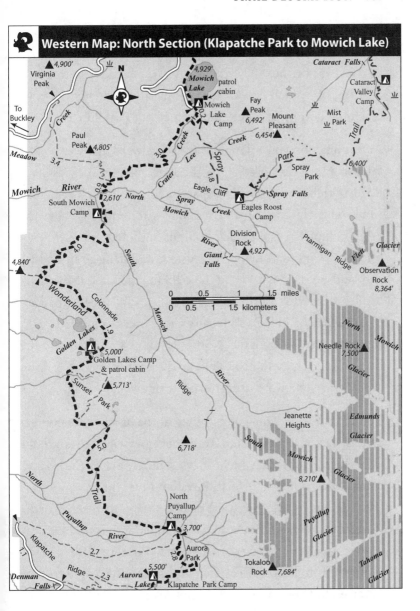

Western Map: North Section (Klapatche Park to Mowich Lake)

From Klapatche Park Camp the trail wanders gently downhill through beautiful subalpine meadows for 0.2 mile and then begins a long downhill. The descent is often steep, so watch your footing. The first 16 irregularly spaced switchbacks take you down to a relatively open area called Aurora Park, where you have good views to the east of the cliffs, spires, and buttes around Tokaloo Rock. Below this point you remain mostly in forest for the next 22 switchbacks, which take you to a log crossing of a small creek. After a final five switchbacks you reach the bottom at a junction with North Puyallup Trail.

At this junction you will notice low stone walls that were built for decorative purposes along the long-abandoned Westside Road. Originally planned as part of a scenic highway that would entirely encircle the mountain, the gravel road was never completed due to lack of funds and other more urgent priorities. The road then suffered repeated damage in floods and landslides, which forced the NPS to close all but the first 3 miles to private cars (though NPS vehicles still use the road as far as Klapatche Ridge). The road's final 3 miles from Klapatche Ridge to just beyond the North Puyallup River have been closed to all vehicles since 1989, and that section of road is now used as the somewhat-overgrown North Puyallup Trail.

The Wonderland Trail goes straight at the junction. It immediately passes a short spur trail that goes right to a stone wall–lined overlook, which offers a nice view of the rocky defile down which the North Puyallup River flows, as well as the cliffs and spires around Tokaloo Rock. To reach North Puyallup Camp, continue on the Wonderland Trail down to a wooden bridge that crosses the North Puyallup River above a short but boisterous waterfall and soon after come to the lower end of the camp. The campsites are spread out along the trail as the route crosses the wooded hillside on the north side of the river. **Tip:** Because these tent sites are located along the shoulder of the old gravel road, they are often quite rocky. It may be difficult to get a tent stake into the ground, so a freestanding tent will work better here.

The old road ends shortly after North Puyallup Camp, after which the rolling trail gains very little elevation over the next mile as you cross a heavily forested hillside. You then round the crest of a minor ridge, and the ascent becomes steeper and more noticeable. Soon after this, you begin going in and out of an old burn that ravaged much of the vicinity in 1930. A few silvery snags are still visible, but the main lingering effects of the blaze are the open terrain and the abundant blueberries, bear grass, and other sunshine-loving plants that have colonized the area. In July of favorable years the bear grass puts on a wonderful show of tall white blossoms, while the berries typically ripen in late August and early September, providing wonderful eating for hikers and black bears alike. On the downside, there is limited shade, which can make the climb hot on summer afternoons. Water is common, however, as you cross plank bridges over several small creeks along the way. About 3.6 miles from North Puyallup Camp, and 0.5 mile after crossing the second of two larger creeks, you hit the top of a rounded ridge.

SIDE TRIP ALERT:
SUNSET PARK VIEWPOINT

From the top of the ridge a sketchy old trail heads northeast across the mostly open slopes of an area known as Sunset Park. The abandoned route leads to one of the finest (but least visited) viewpoints in Mount Rainier National Park, so it's worth seeking out. The tread is initially very faint, but if you head generally uphill and to the north-northeast, you should see pieces of the trail on the hillside above you. The route is inter-mittent, with areas that are fairly overgrown and others that are clear and obvious. The old trail switchbacks up a bear grass–covered hillside, and then climbs less steeply to a meadow near a saddle in the ridge, about 1.1 miles from the Wonderland Trail. Here you are treated to a stupendous view over the deep chasm of the South Mowich River to the bulky west face of Mount Rainier. In early summer a small and very shallow snowmelt pond provides picture-postcard reflections of the mountain. While soaking in the scene, be on the lookout for black bears, which are common along the ridge. From this viewpoint, you can either head back the way you came or follow the old trail as it makes a rounded turn to the west, gradually descends along the top of another ridge to an old fire lookout site, and then drops steeply to the Wonderland Trail. You reunite with the Wonderland Trail at a minor ridgetop, just north of a small creek, about 0.9 mile north of where you left the maintained trail.

The Wonderland Trail goes straight (north) from the first unsigned junction with the abandoned trail to the ridge above Sunset Park and travels up and down past small ponds and through open forest and meadows to the hop-over crossing of a small creek. Less than 0.1 mile after the creek, you round the top of a minor ridge where you might see faint traces of the sketchy trail that heads east up to the great viewpoint atop the ridge above Sunset Park discussed above. You keep straight, gradually descend through mostly open terrain, and then go down three quick switchbacks to a junction less than 30 yards from the Sunset Park/Golden Lakes Patrol Cabin on your left. The quaint log structure has a pleasant setting right above a pretty little lake. To reach Golden Lakes Camp, follow the short path that starts beside the patrol cabin and goes west. Both black bears and mosquitoes are common here, so camp and act accordingly. There are several larger forest-rimmed lakes in the Golden Lakes cluster about 400 feet lower in elevation and northwest of the camp, but they can be reached only by cross-country travel.

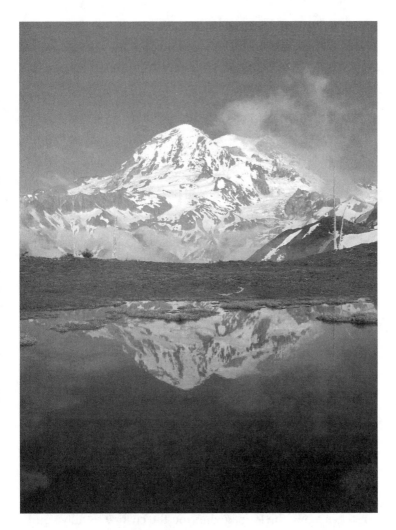

Mount Rainier and snowmelt pond in Sunset Park

From the patrol cabin the Wonderland Trail goes up and down through open forest and past a series of small ponds (also known as mosquito nurseries). The trail then curves to the northwest and goes gradually downhill along the southwest side of Colonnade Ridge. At about 1.5 miles from the patrol cabin the trail breaks out of the forest and enters sloping meadows with lots of wildflowers, including bear grass, lupines, tiger lilies, and pink heather. The ridge provides nice views to the south over the basin holding the Golden Lakes. At 1.9 miles from Golden Lakes the trail tops the ridge and begins to drop down its north side.

SIDE TRIP ALERT: KNOLL 4,840

From the point where the trail drops over the top of Colonnade Ridge, an unsigned but obvious trail, actually an old fire road that is now mostly overgrown, goes west-northwest along the ridgetop. If you follow the route for 0.35 mile, you'll come to the park boundary near the top of an unnamed 4,840-foot knoll. A very short scramble takes you to the top of the knoll, which is covered with grasses and wildflowers. From this grandstand you'll enjoy an exceptionally photogenic view of the Mount Rainier (your last for several miles). You can also look west to the Puget Sound lowlands and the distant Olympic Mountains.

On the north side of Colonnade Ridge the Wonderland Trail abruptly reenters forest and begins a long switchbacking descent. Here begins one of the more extended forested stretches along the loop, giving you the chance to fully appreciate this viewless but perpetually green environment. You will find that unlike the subalpine meadows with their tapestry of colors, forest wildflowers are mostly a demure white or faded pink. Look for foamflowers, vanilla leaf plants, queencups, bunchberries, pipsissewas, twinflowers, starflowers, and baneberries, among others. All of these blossoms are mostly white, but they have distinctive shapes and sizes that make them endlessly interesting and attractive. In addition to the wildflowers, the forest floor is liberally covered with a lush variety of ground cover species, including Oregon grapes, devil's clubs, salals, elderberries, salmonberries, thimbleberries, huckleberries, and at least three types of ferns: deer, sword, and lady. As you lose elevation, the songs of forest birds and the rush of wind rustling the treetops is gradually replaced by the sound of the cascading waters of the South Mowich River. (There is also the frequent buzz of flies and mosquitoes, but let's not dwell on the negative.)

Mount Rainier from Knoll 4,840 northwest of Golden Lakes

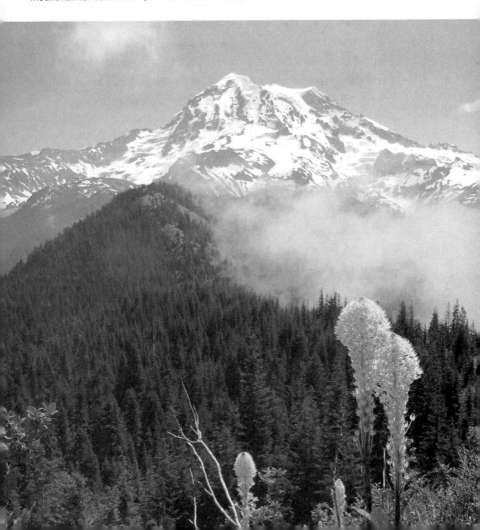

A total of 35 well-graded switchbacks (plus a few rounded twists and turns) lead you down from the high country, dropping a total of 1,900 feet to the valley floor. At the bottom, the trail meanders along, gradually losing a bit of elevation for 0.2 mile to a set of seasonal log bridges spanning the (usually) multiple branches of the silty South Mowich River. The wide riverbed provides one of the few chances for a large opening in the forest cover, allowing good vistas to the north of the heavily forested slopes of Paul Peak and southeast to the snowy crags around Needle Rock and the Jeanette Heights.

About 0.2 mile beyond the river crossing is a junction with a signed spur trail that goes a short distance left to South Mowich Camp. The pleasantly shady spot features a cozy wooden shelter, but it is a fairly long walk back up the way you came to find clear water because the South Mowich River is usually too silt-laden for easy filtering and drinking.

The Wonderland Trail continues straight from the South Mowich Camp junction, still crossing the valley floor beneath

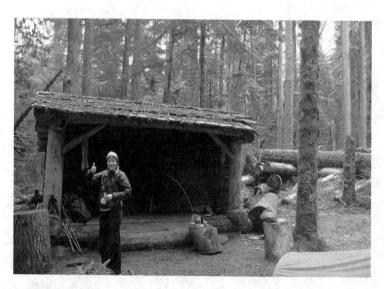

Shelter at South Mowich Camp

the shade of old-growth western red cedars and western hemlocks. After about 0.3 mile you come to the narrow log bridge over similarly silt-laden North Mowich River and then ascend two widely spaced switchbacks to a junction with the lightly used Paul Peak Trail.

You turn sharply right and for the next 3 miles climb the heavily forested slopes on the southeast side of Paul Peak. The ascent is a mix of switchbacks and longer traverses, most of it at a steady, moderately steep grade. Trees obstruct the views, but shade is abundant, which is a blessing on a warm summer afternoon. About 2.6 miles into the climb you approach cascading Crater Creek, which flows out of Mowich Lake. After following this joyful stream for 0.2 mile you cross its flow on a log bridge. Just above the crossing is a wide and very photogenic sliding waterfall that is worth admiring, if only as an excuse to rest after the long climb. Above the crossing you make one more switchback and reach an important junction.

The Spray Park Trail goes to the right. This scenic alternate trail is actually more popular with loop hikers than the official Wonderland Trail because it passes near impressive Spray Falls, visits beautiful Spray and Seattle Parks, and takes you through many miles of wonderful meadows with outstanding flower fields and great viewpoints. Early in the season, however, the exposed, high-elevation trail is usually snow-covered and hard to follow. In addition, if the weather is bad and your permit has your next scheduled campsite at Carbon River, then you are much better off taking the official Wonderland Trail, which stays lower in elevation and is protected by forest for most of the way. Even if you plan to take the Spray Park Trail, you might want to make a quick side trip to Mowich Lake to see the pleasant lake and/or pick up a food cache. To reach the lake, go left at the junction, staying on the

Wonderland Trail, and ascend through forest on a couple of switchbacks for 0.2 mile.

The trail reaches Mowich Lake on the east side of a bridge that connects to a gravel parking lot. Immediately on your right are a small walk-in campground, a restroom, and a sometimes-occupied ranger's patrol cabin. (Food caches sent to this location are left behind the patrol cabin.) Backpackers can stay at the campground, but they must share the facilities with walk-in car campers, which makes it less appealing for hikers. On the positive side, the campground has trash cans, so you can reduce your pack weight by getting rid of any accumulated garbage. In addition, Mowich Lake itself, the largest body of water in Mount Rainier National Park, is quite attractive, especially when you're looking across the clear waters to the rugged heights of Fay Peak and Mother Mountain. You can swim in the lake, if you don't mind cold water, and fishing is also possible, though success rates are low.

Section 2

Mowich Lake to Carbon River Camp Junction via the Wonderland Trail

DISTANCE.. 8.0 miles

Though the majority of loop hikers skip this section, opting instead for the more scenic Spray Park alternative, this pleasant but overlooked section of the Wonderland Trail takes you through some of the oldest and most impressive forests in the park and provides a lower-elevation option when the Spray Park Trail is still buried under several feet of snow.

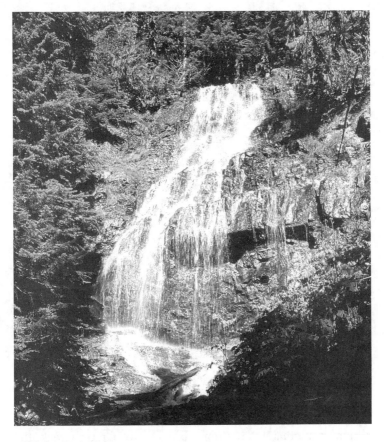

Falls below Eunice Lake

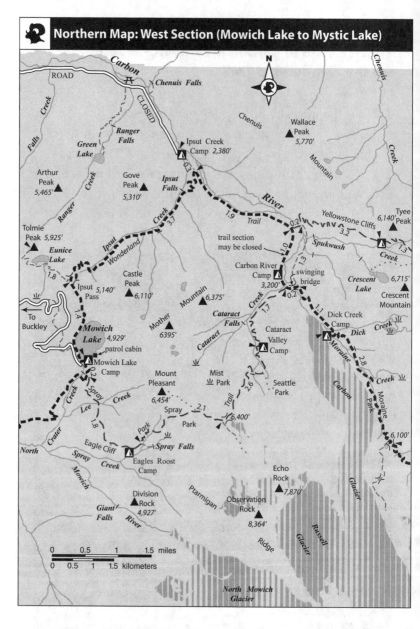

Northern Map: West Section (Mowich Lake to Mystic Lake)

From the campground at Mowich Lake, the trail goes clockwise around the lake, initially hugging the south shore and almost immediately crossing a bridge over Crater Creek, the lake's outlet. On the other side of the bridge is a junction with a short path that leads 15 yards up to the parking lot at the end of a gravel road. Keep straight and continue along the mostly level path that follows a course between the gravel road on the left and the lakeshore on your right. Along the way you will pass several short, unmarked side trails going left to the road (ignore 'em) and right to pleasant lakeshore viewpoints (take these!). After 0.6 mile you come to the northwest corner of Mowich Lake where the trail pulls away from the water and climbs briefly over a little ridge. From here the path descends a bit before traversing a hillside covered with bear grass, huckleberries, Douglas firs, and mountain hemlocks. At 1.4 miles from the Mowich Lake Camp you reach a fork in the trail.

SIDE TRIP ALERT:
EUNICE LAKE AND TOLMIE PEAK

A worthy and popular side trail goes left at this junction. The path descends four short switchbacks and then traverses a wooded hillside to a lovely little waterfall. After this, a couple of uphill switchbacks take you to Eunice Lake, 0.6 mile from the Wonderland Trail junction. This good-size lake is backed by the cliffs of Tolmie Peak and is quite attractive. For the best views, continue past the lake, climbing in occasional switchbacks for 1.2 miles to the fire lookout building on the summit of Tolmie Peak. On a clear day you can see almost 100 miles in every direction. The most photogenic scenes are looking southeast down to the shimmering waters of Eunice Lake and up to the snowy ramparts of Mount Rainier.

The Wonderland Trail goes right at the junction and just 60 yards later arrives at Ipsut Pass, where you will find a nice view down into the dark-green canyons of Ipsut Creek and the Carbon River. The trail then uses numerous, mostly short switchbacks to go steeply downhill on a very rocky tread. Initially the descent takes you across a brushy slope with good views of some tall basalt cliffs that rise immediately beside the tread. A little farther down are some nice views to the southeast of aptly named Castle Peak.

After 19 switchbacks you reenter forest and cross several trickling branches at the headwaters of Ipsut Creek. The trail then becomes much gentler as it follows the creek downstream. Along the way you take log bridges over a series of small creeks, none of which have official names. The third of these creeks is especially lovely because you cross it in the middle of a twisting waterfall. The other striking feature here is the forest. These are some of the largest and oldest trees in Mount Rainier National Park, with some having been measured at more than 1,200 years of age. This remarkable longevity is made possible by the unusual fact that fire has not touched the remote valley in several centuries. In particular, look for an immense Alaska yellow cedar (on the left side of the trail) that, until an even larger one was discovered in Olympic National Park, was thought to be the largest specimen of the species in the world.

After following Ipsut Creek for almost 2 miles, the trail descends a wooded hillside on three long switchbacks to a junction just above a small side channel of the milky Carbon River. If you go straight here, in 0.3 mile you will reach Ipsut Creek Camp. The large site was formerly a car campground at the end of the Carbon River Road. With the closure of that often-flooded thoroughfare, however, the campground has been converted into a backpacker's camp. Without the cars, this is a shady, quiet, and comfortable place to spend the night.

The Wonderland Trail goes sharply right at the junction and travels upstream at a gentle grade never far from the braided and rather unsightly rubble- and log-strewn bed of the Carbon River. Perhaps the most interesting thing about this viewless stretch of trail is the vegetation, which is extremely thick and lush, presenting the hiker with more shades of green than Crayola ever dreamed possible. In fact, you are now walking through one of the few inland temperate rain forests in the world. I hope the weather won't be living up to the rain forest designation when you hike through, but because most hikers get at least *some* rain during the course of their circuit around the mountain, this low-elevation area is probably as good a place as any to encounter the wet stuff. After 1.9 miles you reach a junction.

As of late 2010, the official Wonderland Trail, which used to go straight at this junction, was undergoing major reconstruction after heavy landslide and flood damage. In 2011 the new section of trail was washed out *again,* and the National Park Service was considering closing the trail permanently. If the trail is closed (or still under construction) when you make the trip, then you will have to make a detour. In that case, you turn left on the Northern Loop Trail, cross the Carbon River on a log bridge, and then climb briefly to a junction. Hikers taking the Northern Loop Trail instead of the Wonderland Trail across the northern section of the mountain should turn left. Wonderland Trail hikers taking the detour, however, turn right at the junction and follow a trail that crosses the hillside east of the Carbon River. Most of the way is in forest, but there are some pleasant, if unspectacular, views of the Carbon River and its surrounding forested ridges along the way. After 1.3 miles you come to a junction on the east side of a swinging suspension bridge where you reconnect with the official/old Wonderland Trail. If you are scheduled to stay at Carbon River Camp, then turn right at this junction, cross the narrow suspension bridge, and then walk about 0.2 mile to a junction with Spray Park Trail. Here you turn right, almost immediately cross Cataract Creek, and about 150 yards later reach the camp. If you had to take the detour, then the old Wonderland Trail will likely be closed just north of the camp.

If the Wonderland Trail has been reopened and reconstructed, then go straight at the junction with the detour route, staying on the west side of the Carbon River, and follow this route, which snakes along a rocky and wooded hillside above the rampaging river. After 0.9 mile you reach Carbon River Camp, a popular and very nice camp with good water from nearby Cataract Creek. Just 0.1 mile past Carbon River Camp, and almost immediately after you cross Cataract Creek, is a junction with the Spray Park Trail, the highly scenic alternative to the official Wonderland Trail between Mowich Lake and here.

Section 3

Mowich Lake to Carbon River Camp Junction via the Spray Park Trail

DISTANCE. . . . . 8.4 miles

Though it's not the official Wonderland Trail, most hikers doing the loop around the mountain prefer to use the Spray Park Trail as an alternate way of reaching Carbon River. This is a reasonable choice because the scenery is extremely dramatic and is certainly more impressive than that found along

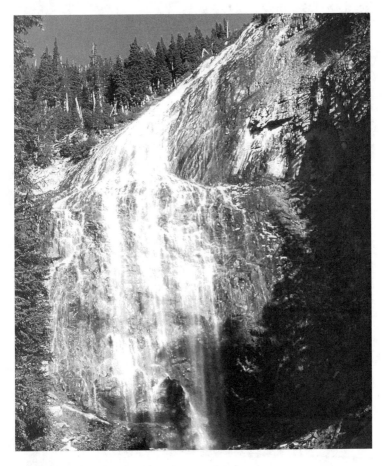

Spray Falls

the actual Wonderland Trail. The main reasons *not* to take this alternative are that it is somewhat more exposed and strenuous, with a couple of miles that are above timberline and an additional 500 feet in elevation gain, and that until as late as mid-August much of the high country near the divide above Spray Park will still be covered with large snowfields. Thus, hikers coming through in July or during inclement weather are better off taking the official Wonderland Trail. Anyone hiking in good weather and a bit later in the summer, however, should opt for the Spray Park alternative and be ready to take lots of pictures.

The Spray Park Trail begins 0.2 mile south of Mowich Lake at the junction with the Wonderland Trail coming up from North Mowich River. Thus, hikers coming from Longmire can either forgo a visit to Mowich Lake and turn directly onto the Spray Park Trail, or make the short side trip to Mowich Lake (to either spend the night or pick up a food cache) before returning to the Spray Park junction.

In either case, you go southeast from the junction onto the Spray Park Trail and begin a series of very minor ups and downs through an attractive midelevation forest. Along the way you make a log crossing of two branches of clear Lee Creek in a wildflower-filled glade. At about 1.4 miles from the junction you come to a signed side trail that goes to the right.

> ## SIDE TRIP ALERT: EAGLE CLIFF
>
> Don't miss the 30-yard dead-end spur trail, which goes steeply downhill to a fine viewpoint atop Eagle Cliff. The scene looking across the deep valley of Spray Creek up to the ice-covered ramparts of Mount Rainier is the best view of the peak you have enjoyed since before Golden Lakes. In 1898 early climber Israel Cook Russell, using

the flowery language of his time, described this spot as having "one of the most sublime pictures of noble scenery to be had anywhere in America." Today we are more likely to say something like "awesome, man," but either does the job admirably.

The main trail goes straight at the turnoff to the Eagle Cliff viewpoint and contours across a forested hillside well above the steep drop-off of Eagle Cliff. Almost 0.4 mile from the viewpoint turnoff is another junction, this time with a trail that goes sharply right and downhill. The 0.1-mile spur trail leads to comfortable, but viewless, Eagles Roost Camp. Because camping is prohibited in Spray Park, this is the last legal campsite before you climb over the high pass ahead.

The Spray Park Trail goes straight at the Eagles Roost turnoff and continues 0.2 mile through forest to yet another junction.

SIDE TRIP ALERT: SPRAY FALLS

Be sure to set aside 30 minutes to make the side trip that goes to the right here to Spray Falls. The trail is just more than 0.2 mile and ends at a rocky area on Spray Creek not far below the wide veil of dramatic Spray Falls. At approximately 280 feet, this is one of the highest waterfalls in the park, and it is quite a sight. The name is descriptive and easy to understand as you'll need to protect yourself and your camera from the abundant water droplets that spread from the falls. On a hot afternoon the spray is quite refreshing. The best views are from the opposite side of the creek, but getting there requires a possibly wet crossing over slippery boulders, so be careful.

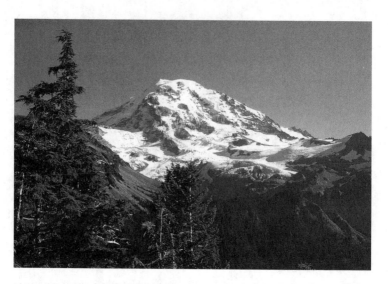

Mount Rainier from Eagle Cliff viewpoint

Back on the Spray Park Trail you rapidly ascend 12 switch-backs before finally breaking out of forest, crossing a log over a small creek, and entering the lower end of the meadows at Spray Park. The views start off with a bang, as straight ahead of you is a wonderful perspective of Mount Rainier, which from this angle has a more slender and refined profile than the bulky mass displayed from other points around the mountain. The trail now ascends through partial forest and increasingly large meadows that provide ever-improving views of the mountain. Several unmarked but obvious side trails branch off to knolls, tiny ponds, or private wildflower glades that are perfect for quiet contemplation away from the crowds of day hikers that visit the area. The trail itself includes countless erosion-barrier "steps," making it seem that you are ascending a long staircase. If your visit is in late July, you may encounter enormous fields of white-blooming avalanche lilies, for which Spray Park is famous.

As the trail continues to gain elevation, the trees get smaller and less numerous, allowing for even better mountain views. Possible side trips, including the tough but fun scramble to the top of Mount Pleasant to the northwest, abound. Remember to hang your pack before doing any major exploring, however, because bears and chipmunks are common and won't hesitate to steal your food. Eventually you pass a particularly fetching little pond on your left with a supremely photogenic view of Mount Rainier, and then leave virtually all the trees behind and climb into a land of alpine meadows and rocks.

You top the divide at an elevation of about 6,400 feet, where large snowfields often cover the trail. To aid in navigation, look for small cairns marking the route, often topped with rocks that have been painted bright red or orange. Before August, however, these navigational aids remain buried, so look for small red flags, which are put in by helpful National Park Service crews. Though it takes considerable effort to get here, the view from the top of the ridge makes the effort worthwhile. In the distance to the north are the rugged peaks of the Alpine Lakes Wilderness, while closer at hand is jagged Mother Mountain. Dominating the scene, however, is the imposing figure of Mount Rainier close by to the southeast. Even this angle's relatively slimmed-down mountain remains incredibly impressive as it rises fully 8,000 feet above your current location.

SIDE TRIP ALERT: UPPER SPRAY PARK

Once at the ridgetop many hikers feel an overwhelming urge to see more and go higher. Fortunately, an obvious boot trail that goes southeast up the adjacent ridge invites you to do just that. Giving in to this exploring urge will be rewarded with lovely hidden ponds, alpine rock gardens, and otherworldly views. The exploring can go on as long as time and ambition allow, but I recommend scheduling at least two hours for poking around and really enjoying the scenery.

The Spray Park Trail descends from the ridge through a land of rocks, grasses, and snowfields, requiring careful attention to the small cairns that mark the circuitous route. After about 0.5 mile you enter friendlier terrain as you pass above the flat and inviting expanse of Mist Park. As you descend further, the landscape continues to soften with lots of heather meadows, small ponds, and scattered trees, offering lovely foregrounds to the views of Crescent Mountain to the east and rugged Mother Mountain to the northwest. The trail wanders down through the flower fields of Seattle Park, passes beside a small waterfall, and then reaches an easy-to-miss junction with a boot path that angles off to the right. This route, which takes explorers over a rocky ridge and into the upper reaches of Seattle Park, is worth the effort if you have some extra time.

The main trail continues descending through the meadows in the lower reaches of Seattle Park, paralleling a small creek for a while before reentering forest and beginning a series of downhill switchbacks. Along the way you pass a short side trail leading to a small waterfall in a gully on your right. Nearly 1 mile from the lower end of Seattle Park is a signed junction with the spur trail to Cataract Valley Camp. Partly because knees are usually starting to complain about all the downhill and partly because this is the first legal campsite since Eagles Roost, Cataract Valley is a popular place for hikers to spend the night. Like almost all of the park's backcountry campsites, it is attractive and comfortable, so it is a good choice for those ready to relax and process their extremely scenic day coming over from Mowich Lake.

Past Cataract Valley Camp the Spray Park Trail, now studded with hundreds of log and stone steps, descends more than two dozen fairly steep switchbacks. At the bottom of these switchbacks the trail parallels mostly unseen Cataract

Creek for 0.6 mile to a junction with the Wonderland Trail. If you turn left here, you will cross Cataract Creek and reach Carbon River Camp in 0.1 mile. The trail that continues north from the camp was formerly (and may be again in the future) the official Wonderland Trail, but repeated flooding and washouts have closed the trail indefinitely as of 2011.

Section 4

Carbon River Camp Junction to Sunrise via the Wonderland Trail

DISTANCE .... 15.1 miles

The Wonderland Trail across the north side of Mount Rainier is varied, dramatic, and often spectacularly beautiful. It includes up-close and personal looks at two rock-covered glaciers, a gorgeous mountain lake, three high passes, lots of wildlife, and the usual flower-covered meadows and views. As if that weren't enough, there are also some excellent side trips to jaw-dropping beauty spots just a short walk off the main trail. The price for all these glories (yes, there's always a price) is two long and steep uphill sections of trail, mosquitoes and bears around Mystic Lake, and snowfields in early summer around Skyscraper Pass. In good weather, almost every hiker agrees that the price is worth paying.

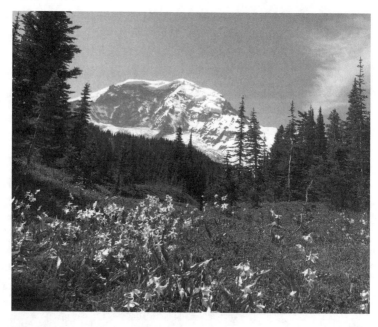

Mount Rainier over lower end of Moraine Park

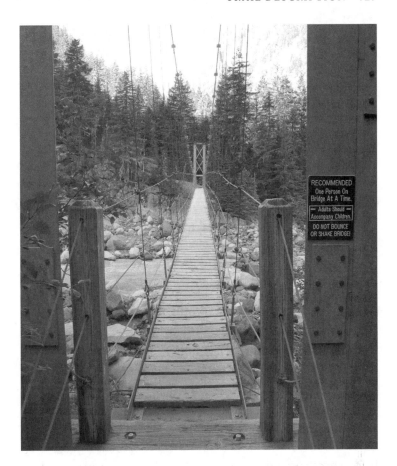

East end of Carbon River bridge

From the junction of the Spray Park and Wonderland Trails just south of Carbon River Camp, you go east and travel about 0.2 mile through forest to the Carbon River suspension bridge. Like the similar span across Tahoma Creek, this structure is very impressive with its tall metal towers and cable-suspended wooden plank surface. The swaying and bouncing motion you endure as you cross (one hiker at a time, please) is unsettling, but it's still a fun and memorable experience. If you took the Wonderland Trail over Ipsut Pass and were forced into the detour up the east side of the Carbon River, then your route will no longer cross the bridge. It's worth a side trip to do it anyway, however, just for the bouncing fun of it!

Immediately on the east side of the bridge is a junction. Hikers heading for the Northern Loop Trail alternative turn left here (see the description in the next section), but Wonderland Trail hikers go right (upstream) and soon begin one of the longest and steepest climbs along the entire Wonderland Trail. You will gain 2,900 feet in 3.6 miles, with only a few relatively level stretches to give your tired muscles a break. So settle in for a long haul and set off through a pleasant forest. You soon leave the trees and climb a very steep and rocky route on the slopes adjoining Carbon Glacier, the lowest-elevation glacier in the continental United States. A sign correctly warns you to stay off the rock-covered ice due to the extreme danger of cave-ins, ice- and rockfalls, swift water, and crevasses. **Tip:** The trail beside the glacier is fully exposed to the afternoon sun, so try to do this section in the cool of the morning.

A detour that uses two switchbacks to circumvent a washout provides a short respite from the steep uphill, but the steepness soon resumes as it charges up the rocky slope to a log bridge over cascading Dick Creek. Just beyond the crossing is tiny Dick Creek Camp. The camp is located atop a rock outcrop almost directly overlooking the ice of Carbon Glacier.

The trail continues its steep uphill with 11 switchbacks, most of which are, thankfully, in the shade of a forest, leading to a lacy waterfall on a small, unnamed side creek. You then ascend at a more gradual pace following pretty little Moraine Creek for about 0.5 mile. With the added elevation you soon start to enter subalpine meadows with abundant wildflowers. Four more short switchbacks and an uphill meander take you to the lovely rolling meadow at Moraine Park. There is a very nice view of Mount Rainier, as well as good looks of

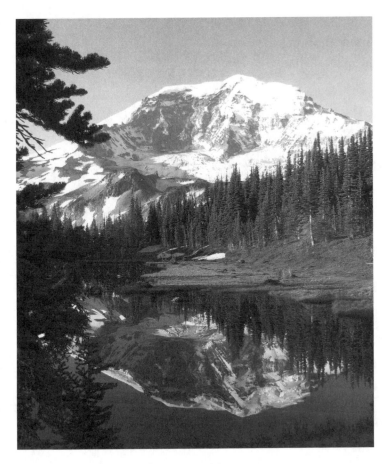

Mount Rainier and tarn at pass above Mystic Lake

Ptarmigan Ridge to the southwest from the lower (north) end of the grassy meadow. Sharing the view is a large population of hoary marmots. These cute, furry, housecat-size critters are probably more abundant here than anywhere else along the Wonderland Trail. Above Moraine Park you ascend 10 more steep switchbacks before finally finishing the long uphill at a 6,100-foot pass.

A shallow tarn on the right (west) side of the trail offers outstanding views across its water to towering Willis Wall and the overwhelming north face of Mount Rainier. On a still morning the reflection of the mountain in this tarn is breathtaking.

SIDE TRIP ALERT: WILLIS WALL VIEWPOINT

Adventurous hikers won't want to miss a wonderful side trip from the pass. Look for an unmaintained but easy-to-follow use trail that goes around the tarn and then climbs to the south. The path leads to a stunning up-close view of Willis Wall from the moraine above the head of Carbon Glacier. You pass one excellent viewpoint after only 0.8 mile, but if you're still feeling spry, you can continue the journey by dropping to a saddle and then climbing for another 1.2 miles on this wildly scenic route before it finally becomes too steep and rocky for most hikers. **Tip:** Photographers will need a *super* wide-angle lens to capture the enormity of the scenes that unfold along the upper parts of the trail.

Back at the pass, you descend five switchbacks to an idyllic little valley and then go over a minor secondary ridge before arriving at the tranquil meadow-rimmed shore of Mystic Lake. Old Desolate Mountain provides a fine backdrop to the scene, rising above the north side of the lake. To the south, Mineral Mountain blocks the view of Mount Rainier, though you can get a partial look at it from near the patrol cabin on the northeast side of the lake.

The trail rounds the south side of Mystic Lake, passes a side trail to the Mystic Patrol Cabin, and then goes downhill for 0.2 mile to the turnoff to Mystic Camp. This is a popular overnight stop for backpackers, and the local bruins have

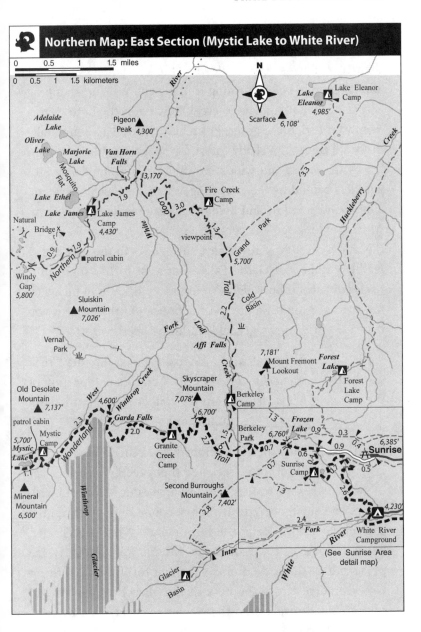

Northern Map: East Section (Mystic Lake to White River)

0   0.5   1   1.5 miles
0   0.5   1   1.5 kilometers

N

Adelaide Lake
Oliver Lake
Pigeon Peak 4,300'
Scarface 6,108'
Lake Eleanor 4,985'
Lake Eleanor Camp

Marjorie Lake
Van Horn Falls
3,170'
1.9
3.0
Loop
3.3
Fire Creek Camp

Lake Ethel
Lake James
Lake James Camp 4,430'
viewpoint
Grand Park
5,700'

Natural Bridge X
1.9
patrol cabin
1.3
2.2
Cold Basin

Windy Gap 5,800'
Northern
0.9
Sluiskin Mountain 7,026'
White Fork
Lodi Creek
Affi Falls
7,181'
Mount Fremont Lookout
Forest Lake

Vernal Park
West Winthrop Creek
4,600'
Skyscraper Mountain 7,078'
6,700'
Berkeley Camp
Forest Lake Camp

Old Desolate Mountain 7,137'
patrol cabin
5,700'
Mystic Camp
Mystic Lake
2.3
Wonderland
Garda Falls 2.0
Granite Creek Camp
Trail
1.5
Berkeley Park 6,760'
0.7
Frozen Lake 0.9
0.3
0.9
0.4
6,385'
Sunrise

1.1
Mineral Mountain 6,500'
Windthrop Glacier
2.7
2.8
Second Burroughs Mountain 7,402'
0.6
Sunrise Camp
0.7
1.3
0.5
2.6
2.4
Fork
White River
White River Campground

Glacier Basin
Inter
White
(See Sunrise Area detail map)
4,230'

taken notice. Don't be surprised if you see a bear wandering around camp, so be sure to hang your food. Mosquitoes can be a problem here as well.

The trail descends from Mystic Camp through forest for 0.2 mile to a log crossing of clear West Fork White River. You then turn downstream, following the cascading waters for about 0.2 mile before turning to the right and rock-hopping across of a small, unnamed creek flowing in the bottom of a deeply eroded, rocky gorge. From here the trail goes gradually downhill through a shady forest for about 0.3 mile and then leaves the forest and winds its way across a boulder wasteland left behind by the retreating Winthrop Glacier. Heather, alders, and small fir and hemlock trees now live in this area, which not long ago was completely barren. As you hike across this rocky stretch you will have nice views to the east of the feathery ribbon of Garda Falls, southeast to the sharp pinnacles of Second Burroughs Mountain, and south to the wide, icy mass of Mount Rainier. At the bottom of the descent you take a log bridge over glacial Winthrop Creek.

After a 0.1-mile ascent you come to a log over Granite Creek just below cartwheeling Garda Falls. Only a small portion of the tall waterfall is visible from the trail crossing, but it's still a nice spot to rest in the cooling mist.

From Garda Falls the trail climbs beside the loudly cascading waters of Winthrop Creek and then steeply ascends a set of switchbacks on a rocky moraine that is now covered with alders and small evergreens. Below you and on your right is the rubble-strewn ice at the terminus of Winthrop Glacier, the second-largest ice sheet on Mount Rainier. Dirty ice pokes out of the rock, and the rushing torrent of Winthrop Creek emerges from the base of the glacier. As always, do not attempt to walk onto the glacier as rockfalls, crevasses, and icefalls are all common hazards. Rising over the ice is the towering bulk of Mount Rainier.

You pass a particularly good viewpoint of Mount Rainier at a rocky promontory and then make another steep uphill on a sometimes brushy trail. Your tired muscles catch a break for about 0.2 mile as the trail offers a section of gentle ups and downs, but then it's another steep ascent for about 0.5 mile on a heavily wooded hillside. A half-dozen twists and turns masquerading as proper switchbacks have been put in to give the impression that the trail builders weren't completely sadistic, but it's not very convincing. After conquering this steep section you wander gently up and down for 0.3 mile to a log crossing of Granite Creek and, immediately thereafter, reach Granite Creek Camp. Beyond the camp the trail ascends four moderately graded and widely spaced switchbacks as it slowly leaves the forest, enters meadows, and finally tops out on a ridge just above the low point of often-windy Skyscraper Pass. At about 6,700 feet, this is the second-highest point on the Wonderland Trail, so it's not surprising that the views are first rate. Especially noteworthy are Mount Rainier filling the sky to the south and much daintier Skyscraper Mountain standing close by to the north.

SIDE TRIP ALERT:
SKYSCRAPER MOUNTAIN

From the Wonderland Trail just above Skyscraper Pass, an obvious use trail goes north. The path briefly descends to the saddle of the actual pass and then steeply climbs the south ridge of Skyscraper Mountain to its summit. From the top are the expected great views of Mount Rainier, but you can also look north to the flat, green expanse of Grand Park and even into the distance to Glacier Peak and the rugged Alpine Lakes Wilderness. Very lucky hikers might see mountain goats on the slopes of Skyscraper Mountain.

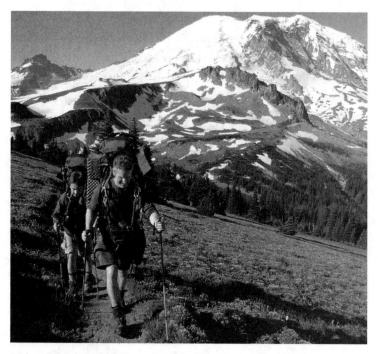

Backpackers approaching Skyscraper Pass

The Wonderland Trail crosses to the west side of the ridge at Skyscraper Pass, rounds a spur ridge just 150 yards later, and then makes a 0.2-mile downhill traverse of an open slope to the rolling meadows in the upper part of Berkeley Park. You pass a good-sized spring and then contour across the meadows to the east end of Berkeley Park. There is a junction here with the Northern Loop Trail, the alternate route across the north side of the mountain.

> **SIDE TRIP ALERT:** BERKELEY PARK POND
>
> From the junction of the Wonderland and Northern Loop Trails, take five minutes to drop your pack and wander about 200 yards north across the trailless tundra to a shallow pond that offers wonderful reflections of the top third of Mount Rainier.

From the junction you bear right (east) on the Wonderland Trail. You gradually ascend through increasingly stark alpine terrain for 0.7 mile to an often windy saddle and a five-way junction not far from aptly named Frozen Lake. The trail to the left ascends then follows a scenic ridge for 1.3 miles to the staffed fire lookout tower on the ridge north of Mount Fremont. The trail that goes sharply to the right climbs to the outstanding viewpoint on the treeless alpine plateau atop First Burroughs Mountain. Straight ahead is an alternate higher-elevation trail for reaching the lodge at Sunrise. This scenic route is probably the better way to go if you are a section hiker and are finishing up at Sunrise. The downside for thru-hikers on the Wonderland Trail, however, is that the higher trail bypasses Sunrise Camp, a convenient overnight location for those doing the loop.

Thru-hikers should go slightly right and downhill at the five-way junction, staying on the Wonderland Trail, and descend

Mount Rainier reflected in pond in Berkeley Park

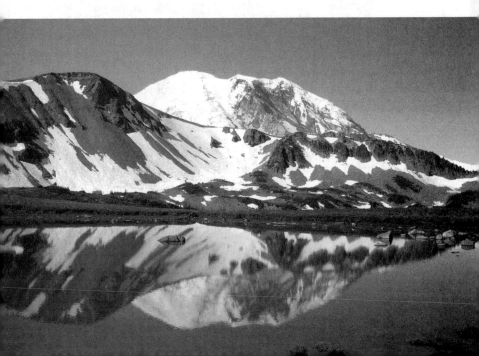

a very rocky and often steep route for 0.6 mile to a junction at the end of a gravel road. The road is closed to private vehicles, so it sees very little use. The shortest route to reach Sunrise—where you can pick up a food cache, shop at the lodge gift shop, or buy a hamburger at the restaurant—is to go straight and walk the gravel road 0.9 mile to the parking lot and lodge. Late-season hikers should note that the lodge, along with its shop and restaurant, closes after Labor Day. Hikers looking to set up camp should go right at the junction and take a meandering route that wanders mostly south for 0.4 mile through meadows and open forest to Sunrise Camp, a pleasant spot not far from small but very pretty Shadow Lake. About 40 yards south of Sunrise Camp is a junction with the Sunrise Rim Trail.

SIDE TRIP ALERT: GLACIER OVERLOOK

Before turning left on the Wonderland Trail, be sure to make a short side trip up the trail to the right, which makes a 0.2-mile uphill traverse to stone wall–lined Glacier Overlook. The view of Mount Rainier and the dirty ice of huge Emmons Glacier far below is unsurpassed. The viewpoint makes a fine destination for a short stroll either in the evening before bed or (better for photography) early in the morning before breakfast.

The Wonderland Trail goes left (east) from the junction just south of Sunrise Camp and soon passes an unsigned side trail that veers left to Shadow Lake. You keep right and wander mostly on the level past Shadow Lake and a wet meadow, cross a small creek, and then walk through open subalpine-fir forests. The views looking southwest back to Mount Rainier are outstanding. After 0.7 mile you come to a junction. The

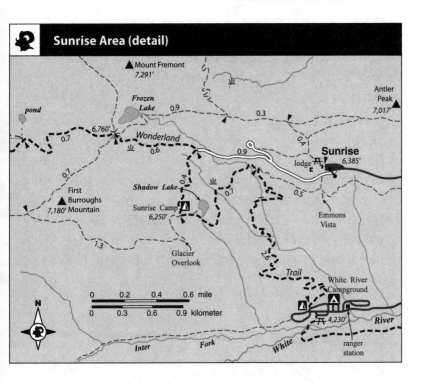

Wonderland Trail goes right. If you are heading to Sunrise, however, go straight and climb gradually through open forests for 0.5 mile to another junction. Here you turn left and in 0.1 mile reach the parking lot at Sunrise Lodge.

Section 5

Carbon River Camp Junction to Berkeley Park and Sunrise via the Northern Loop Trail

DISTANCE...20.7 miles

Hikers who are unable to obtain a permit for the Wonderland Trail across the north side of Mount Rainier need not lose hope of completing the loop. There is a wonderful alternative that is much less popular (and therefore somewhat easier to obtain a permit for) and almost as scenic. Though the Northern Loop Trail is a rugged up-and-down route, it does offer the considerable rewards of lots of wildlife, abundant huckleberries in late summer and early fall, a visit to a pretty

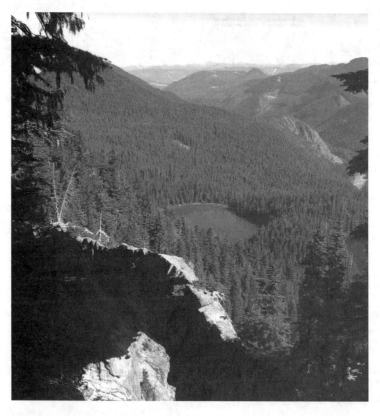

Natural Bridge and Lake Ethel

mountain lake, the chance to explore the very scenic meadow at Grand Park, and a side trip to a huge natural bridge. The route is most often done as part of a spectacular three- to five-day loop trip that starts at Sunrise and combines the Northern Loop Trail with a return along the Wonderland Trail. In fact, for hikers who love loops but who don't have the time or inclination to do the entire Wonderland Trail, this is an excellent shorter alternative. The other possible reason to choose the Northern Loop Trail instead of the Wonderland is that it is somewhat lower in elevation, so through July, when snow still blankets parts of the official Wonderland Trail, the Northern Loop Trail is usually snow free and hikeable.

As previously mentioned, there are two approaches to the western end of the Northern Loop Trail, depending on which route you took over the divide from Mowich Lake. If you hiked the official Wonderland Trail via Ipsut Pass and Carbon River, you will reach the Northern Loop Trail junction 1.9 miles up the trail from the turnoff to Ipsut Creek Campground. If, on the other hand, you hiked the Spray Park Trail over from Mowich Lake, you can best reach the Northern Loop Trail by walking 0.9 mile down the Wonderland Trail from Carbon River Camp along the west side of the Carbon River, assuming this often-damaged section of trail is open when you are there. In either case, you turn east at the Northern Loop Trail junction and walk through a rubble-strewn riverbed to a series of log bridges across the ever-shifting branches of the braided Carbon River. After completing the crossing, the trail ascends a couple of quick switchbacks and comes to a junction. The Northern Loop Trail goes to the left.

If you hiked over via Spray Park, and the Wonderland Trail on the west side of the Carbon River is closed, then you must make a detour to reach this junction. In this case, you cross the Carbon River on the swinging suspension bridge 0.2 mile southeast of Carbon River Camp, and then turn left (north) immediately on the east side of the river and follow the trail for 1.3 miles to the previously mentioned junction with the Northern Loop Trail.

The Northern Loop Trail goes north at the junction and shortly after begins a long uphill. The ascent is relentless with a seemingly endless series of moderately steep and waterless switchbacks that steadily take you up the slopes of Chenuis Mountain. The forest here has very little undergrowth, but the canopy provides lots of shade for tired hikers. After 21 switchbacks the grade eases and you climb at a more gradual pace through a series of small meadows. Eventually you come to a large sloping meadow that is directly beneath the impressive cliffs and spires of the Yellowstone Cliffs. The meadow hosts the Yellowstone Cliffs Camp, a nice spot to either spend the night or at least replenish your depleted water supply in the nearby creek. At a minimum you will want to take a moment to rest and enjoy the area's diverse vegetation, which includes lots of bear grass, huckleberries, heather, and various wildflowers.

From Yellowstone Cliffs Camp a dozen more switchbacks lead up through increasingly gorgeous meadows to Windy Gap, right under the bulky mass of Crescent Mountain. There are sparkling tarns here on both sides of the trail and lots of worthwhile exploring. One excellent route goes north past two ponds to a pass and ridge with great views, including the top part of Mount Rainier. A second outstanding, but usually overlooked, side trip starts at the west end of the largest pond just on the west side of Windy Gap and goes west-southwest, following a sketchy boot path around a ridge and then dropping to deep and scenic Crescent Lake.

On the east side of Windy Gap the trail descends for 0.15 mile to a signed junction.

SIDE TRIP ALERT: NATURAL BRIDGE

The trail to the left is a fun side trip that should not be missed. The 0.9-mile one-way route follows a gentle course over rocky areas and through meadows for the first 0.7 mile, and then rapidly descends 10 short switchbacks to a dramatic viewpoint a little above the large rock arch that carries the descriptive, but rather unimaginative, name of Natural Bridge. It is hard to photograph this geologic landmark, but the view past the arch down to clear Lake James and greenish Lake Ethel is very nice. Sadly, in the distance you can also see several clear-cut scars on US Forest Service land outside of the park.

Back on the Northern Loop Trail you descend through rolling meadowland that offers not only terrific views of the nearby crags of Crescent and Sluiskin Mountains but also some of the greatest concentrations of huckleberries in the park. If you are hiking through from mid-August to mid-September, be prepared for a feast. Also keep in mind that all those berries attract black bears, which are often encountered here during the same period. At the bottom of the meadows you cross a small creek and then begin a series of two dozen moderately steep switchbacks that descend a forested hillside. Eventually you reach a signed junction with a 0.2-mile spur trail to the Lake James Patrol Cabin. Keep straight on the main trail and descend four more switchbacks to the meadows, small inlet creeks, and forests around Lake James. At a prominent turn in the trail, an obvious but unsigned spur trail goes left to a nice spot on the southwest shore of Lake James. The shallow and tranquil lake is surrounded by forested ridges and has no mountain views but is still very pretty. The main trail goes right at the unsigned junction and travels 150 yards to the signed turnoff with the spur trail that goes left to Lake James

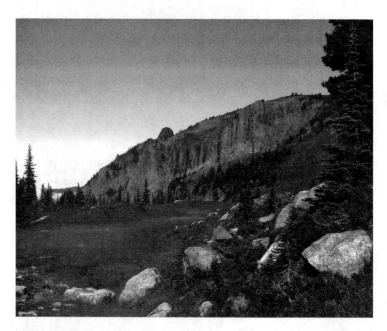

Yellowstone Cliffs from Windy Gap

Camp. **Tip:** Lake James sits at the south end of a forested bench that includes several other lakes to the north. These lakes can be reached by determined hikers who are willing to bushwhack, but be prepared: this bench carries the rather ominous name of Mosquito Flat.

After leaving the peaceful environs of Lake James, the Northern Loop Trail charges downhill, steeply losing elevation in some 25 mostly short switchbacks. There are no views along the way, but the forest provides welcome shade. At the bottom of the descent the path abruptly levels off near a nice resting spot just before a log bridge across the main stem of silt-laden West Fork White River. Just before you cross, however, take the time to visit pretty Van Horn Falls, which you can hear on the side creek immediately to your left (north). **Warning:** When scrambling up to the falls, beware of tangles of devil's club, a nasty plant with many sharp thorns along its stem and below the plant's large leaves.

After crossing West Fork White River you reenter forest and soon come to an unsigned but obvious junction with an abandoned trail that goes left (downstream). You turn right and for the next 0.5 mile slowly gain elevation as you parallel the river and hike past dozens of large downed logs. At the end of this section you pull away from the water and begin the next tough uphill. Using 22 irregularly spaced and moderately steep switchbacks you climb 1,700 feet in the next 2.5 miles to the signed junction with the spur trail to Fire Creek Camp. This viewless but well-located camp, which is 0.35 mile down the dead-end side trail, has two shady tent sites and reliable water from a tiny creek.

The Northern Loop Trail goes right at the Fire Creek Camp turnoff and continues climbing another 13 moderately steep switchbacks before coming to a stunning viewpoint at the top of a rocky cliff. From here you have an extremely photogenic view of Mount Rainier and Sluiskin Mountain rising over the

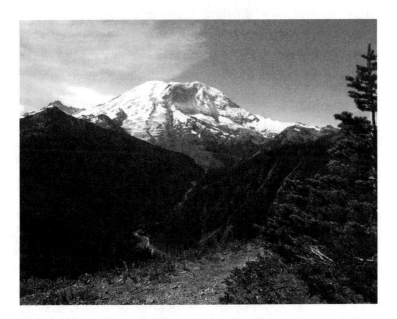

Mount Rainier from viewpoint west of Grand Park

immense depths of the canyon of West Fork White River. **Warning:** Don't get too close to the edge here because the rocks are unstable.

The climb ends soon after the viewpoint as you reenter forest and then break out of the trees near a junction at the southwest corner of Grand Park. This aptly named place is one of the wonders of Mount Rainier National Park, not only because the huge meadow is very beautiful and offers wonderful views of the park's namesake mountain, but also because in a park where almost all the terrain is steep and rugged, Grand Park is remarkably flat. The meadow sits atop a remnant of a massive old basalt flow that has not yet eroded away to form the usual sharp-edged ridges found elsewhere in the park. The trail that meets your route at this junction goes left (northeast) to Lake Eleanor, 3.3 miles away. The lake isn't spectacular but is quiet and wonderfully remote. Even if you don't visit the lake, it is worth taking the first mile or so of the trail to explore more of the huge expanse of Grand Park. **Tip:** While at the extreme south end of Grand Park, take some time to explore off-trail. About 150 yards east of the main trail is a tiny shallow pond, which offers picture-postcard reflections of Mount Rainier.

The Northern Loop Trail goes straight at the Lake Eleanor junction, briefly skirts the corner of Grand Park, and then climbs a bit over a low knoll before going back downhill into forest. You soon level out not far above hard-to-reach (and not really worth it even if you could) Affi Falls. The trail then follows the banks of lovely Lodi Creek upstream for 0.6 mile to very attractive Berkeley Camp. With its small meadow, lots of wildflowers, and excellent views up to the crags of Skyscraper Mountain, this is a particularly nice spot to spend the night.

Above Berkeley Camp the trail continues climbing along Lodi Creek, gradually exchanging forest cover for large and

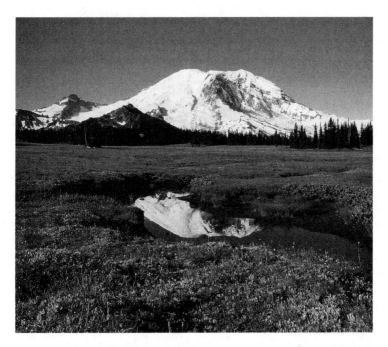

Mount Rainier over Grand Park

attractive meadows. You pass a spring at the head of the creek and then make one long, uphill switchback across an open, wildflower-covered slope to the high basin of Berkeley Park and a reunion with the Wonderland Trail. Keep left and follow the directions to Sunrise given in the previous section that describes the Wonderland Trail.

Section 6

Sunrise to Fryingpan Creek/ Summerland Trailhead

DISTANCE......5.5 miles (including the 0.5 mile from Sunrise Lodge to where you reach the Wonderland Trail)

From a scenery perspective, this short section's highlights are all packed into the first mile as you travel through the famous meadows near Sunrise. The views from here across the deep chasm of the White River and up to Mount Rainier are, along with those from Paradise on the south side of the peak, the most famous views of the mountain. It's truly a photographer's paradise as Rainier displays all of its glory in a massive display of towering height, plunging glaciers, and general mountain grandeur. After leaving the Sunrise area, the trail plunges down a wooded hillside to White River Campground and then parallels roads for 2.4 miles to the popular trailhead at Fryingpan Creek. The main function of this section is to serve as a prelude to your next decision point, where you

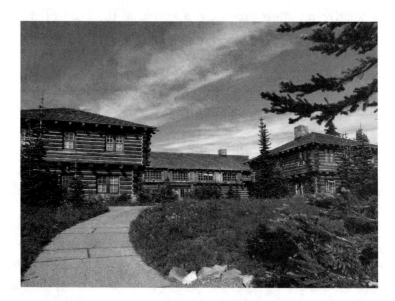

Sunrise Lodge

must pick either the wildly scenic Wonderland Trail over Panhandle Gap or the lower and safer, but less spectacular, Eastside Trail alternative.

Though thru-hikers on the Wonderland Trail will hike in from the west via Sunrise Camp, section hikers will start the route from the northeast at Sunrise Lodge. To reach the Wonderland Trail from there, go south on a path that departs from the south side of the huge parking lot near where a gated gravel road goes to the west. Walk gently downhill for 0.1 mile and then come to a junction. To reach the Wonderland Trail you turn right on the Sunrise Rim Trail.

SIDE TRIP ALERT: EMMONS VISTA

Before heading for the Wonderland Trail, take a few minutes for a side trip that goes straight for 75 yards to Emmons Vista. The view from here, like all those near Sunrise, is awe inspiring and includes a particularly good perspective of Emmons Glacier backed by the pinnacle of Little Tahoma. With luck, and a very strong set of binoculars, you might spot mountain goats on appropriately named Goat Island Mountain, the ridge that rises to the left (southeast) of Emmons Glacier.

After retracing your steps to the junction just north of Emmons Vista, go left (west) on the Sunrise Rim Trail and hike generally downhill through open forest, enjoying frequent views of Mount Rainier. At 0.5 mile from Sunrise you reach a junction with the Wonderland Trail. The trail going straight heads for Sunrise Camp and is how thru-hikers reach this point.

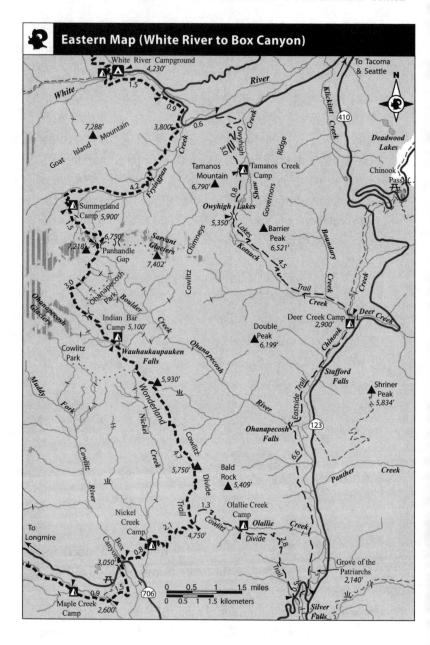

Eastern Map (White River to Box Canyon)

Regardless of how you got there, turn south (downhill) on the Wonderland Trail and begin an extended downhill that loses 1,900 feet in the next 2.6 miles. Though there are a couple of relatively level sections, for the most part it's a consistent, moderately graded descent. A total of 21 switchbacks keep the downhill from being too steep.

During the first four switchbacks you'll have good views of Goat Island Mountain to the south and towering Mount Rainier to the southwest. After this point, however, you cross a small creek in the middle of a tall, cascading waterfall and then enter forest, which allows for only occasional glimpses of the area's famous mountains. Several tiny creeks cross the trail, adding scenic interest, and the forest is pleasantly shady along the wide and easy path. At the bottom is White River Campground. A sign just before you reach the campground's road directs you to the right to the walk-in campsites for

Mount Rainier over White River

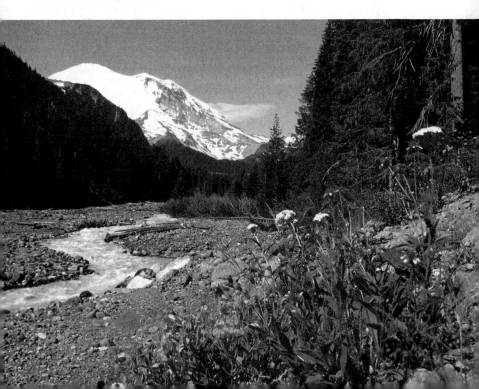

Wonderland Trail hikers (a permit is required). Surrounded by car campers, these campsites do not provide a wilderness experience, but they are conveniently located and well sheltered by the forest. In addition, the campground has piped water, restrooms, and garbage cans where you can throw away your accumulated trash.

At the campground road you go left (east), walk about 50 yards, and then turn in to the day-use hiker parking area on your right. The Wonderland Trail resumes near the restroom building at the west end of the parking lot. *Note:* If you sent a food cache to White River Campground, you will find your supplies behind the ranger station at the lower (east) end of the campground about a 0.1-mile road walk from the day-use parking lot.

The Wonderland Trail goes briefly through a picnic area beside the day-use lot and then crosses the White River on a log bridge amid the usual boulder-strewn wasteland that typifies glacial streams in the park. Looking upstream there is a nice view of about 60% of Mount Rainier. After a very brief detour upstream, the trail curves to the left and heads downstream on the heavily forested hillside and valley floor south of White River. This is a relatively new section of the Wonderland Trail; before 2006, hikers had to walk along the access road to White River Campground to the road bridge over White River. The new trail provides a wilder and much more pleasant hiking experience. After 1.3 miles of mostly level and shady walking, the trail descends for 0.2 mile to a junction with the old Wonderland Trail a little above the White River Road.

You go straight and parallel the road, the occasional traffic noise from which puts a small dent in your wilderness experience. The gentle, woodsy path remains in the forest a little

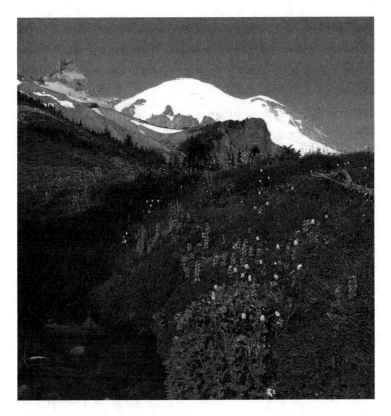

Mount Rainier over creek in Summerland

above the road for 0.9 mile before coming to a junction with a trail that goes left 0.1 mile to the popular Fryingpan Creek/ Summerland Trailhead.

Section 7

Fryingpan Creek/Summerland Trailhead to Box Canyon via the Wonderland Trail

DISTANCE...16.4 miles

On a trail abounding in superlatives, the Wonderland Trail across the east side of Mount Rainier may be the most superb of all. It includes the trip's most abundant wildlife, its highest point, its starkest alpine landscapes, its most numerous waterfalls, two of its prettiest campsites, and, in my opinion, its single most beautiful viewpoint. So what's not to love? Well, early in the season (and often all summer) long stretches of this section are buried under large snowfields, and navigating across them can be a challenge. There is also the concern that in bad weather several miles of the route remain at or above timberline, where you will be dangerously exposed to the cold and wind. But in good weather this rugged section is a hiker's dream, offering a glorious abundance of all the attributes that you probably came to the Wonderland Trail to see. So pray to the weather gods and hope they grace your journey with clear skies and warm temperatures so that you can fully appreciate this magnificent section's countless charms.

From the junction 0.1 mile above the Fryingpan Creek/ Summerland Trailhead, you follow a wide and heavily used trail that goes very gradually uphill through a mature, shady forest. Not far to your left you can hear, but rarely see, the steady flow of clear Fryingpan Creek. After about 0.7 mile the pace of your ascent picks up noticeably, though it still doesn't qualify as steep. At 1.5 miles from the junction you start a set of four switchbacks. Right below the first switchback is a frothing, stair-step waterfall in a narrow chasm on Fryingpan Creek. Above the switchbacks the steady climb continues unabated as the forest gradually becomes more open, and you begin to gather partial views of Mount Rainier and the tall ridges and peaks on either side of Fryingpan Creek. If you hike through these forests and meadows in September, you will often hear the eerie sound of bugling elk. The unique mating call has been described as resembling the high-pitched squeal of bad truck brakes and seems like an odd sound coming from a large mammal.

At a little less than 3 miles from the White River Road you cross a log bridge over Fryingpan Creek and soon thereafter enter wildflower-covered meadows that offer fine views of the broad, snowy cone of Mount Rainier. The jagged pinnacle rising from the left side of the mountain is Little Tahoma. Geologists believe that the 11,138-foot side peak is

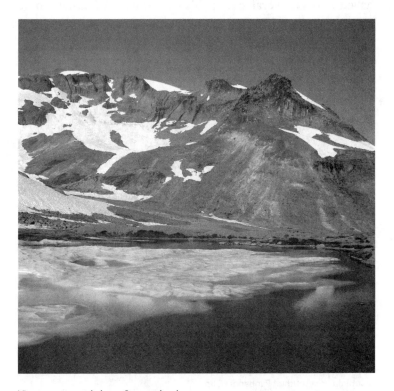

View across pond above Summerland

a remnant of Mount Rainier when it was an even higher and more massive volcano.

The trail now makes nine moderately steep uphill switchbacks before arriving at the famous wildflower-carpeted meadows of Summerland. There is an excellent (and very popular) camp here, including a group site beside a stone shelter.

The Wonderland Trail keeps right at the junction with the spur trail to Summerland Camp, crosses a little creek, and continues going uphill in beautiful meadows and over talus slopes. About 0.3 mile above Summerland you enter what in many years might accurately be called "winter land," an above-timberline region of tiny alpine wildflowers, tufts of grass, fields of rocks, and large snowfields. You will probably have to cross several snowfields over the next 5 miles, so be prepared for icy conditions on cold mornings and wet snow crawling over the tops of your boots on warm afternoons (unless you remembered those gaiters).

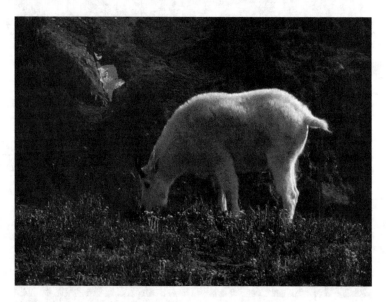

Mountain goat south of Panhandle Gap

You pass a two-tier waterfall on a small creek, cross the creek on a log, and then snake your way uphill through the rugged alpine environment. This area is probably the best place on the Wonderland Trail to see mountain goats, so keep an eye on the nearby rocky cliffs for these amazingly nimble animals. If the snows have melted enough to reveal it, you soon pass a small pond at the base of a semipermanent snowfield. From there the trail winds uphill in twists and turns before finally topping out at Panhandle Gap. At about 6,750 feet this is the highest elevation reached by the Wonderland Trail, so stop to rest and congratulate yourself. The view to the south, especially of the distant Goat Rocks, is inspiring.

SIDE TRIP ALERT:
PANHANDLE GAP BUTTES

Unfortunately, the views of Mount Rainier from Panhandle Gap are mostly blocked by a rocky butte to the west. To rectify this situation, a side trip is in order. For a very short detour, follow a boot path to the left (east) that climbs in less than 0.1 mile nearly to the top of a small knoll with a nice view of the mountain. From there a sketchy but easy-to-navigate route continues east down to a wide saddle, and then up sloping alpine meadows to a 7,402-foot peak directly above the Sarvent Glaciers. From here you have a fine view not only to the west of Mount Rainier but also to the east of the nearby spires of the Cowlitz Chimneys.

Another option from Panhandle Gap is to climb the butte west of the pass. A very steep but obvious boot trail ascends almost to the top of the rugged crags atop the butte, gaining 450 feet in a little less than 0.4 mile. The view from here of Mount Rainier, Little Tahoma, and Fryingpan and Emmons Glaciers is outstanding.

From Panhandle Gap the Wonderland Trail goes south-southwest, initially losing a bit of elevation but then going up and down across a high alpine bench, where you cross rocky slopes and (usually) large snowfields. In foggy or snowy conditions navigation can be especially challenging on this section, so watch carefully for little orange flags and cairns marking the route. After about 1 mile you go past a small pond, which may be iced over all summer, and then do a bit more up and down before topping a minor ridge. From there the trail, which has hundreds of erosion-barrier steps, goes steeply downhill following the top of this little ridge. On your right are excellent views of the cliffs and waterfalls at the head of the deep canyon of the upper Ohanapecosh River. After quickly losing almost 700 feet you come to a saddle.

SIDE TRIP ALERT:
OHANAPECOSH PARK WATERFALLS

If you are an experienced off-trail hiker who loves waterfalls, then take the time for an excellent side trip that begins at the saddle. Go cross-country down the relatively gentle slope on the left (northeast) side of the trail into the rolling meadowlands of Ohanapecosh Park. Once at the bottom, make your way to the base of a long, sliding waterfall that you can see about 0.3 mile away to the north-northeast. You can turn around here, well satisfied, but if you still have the energy, follow a rough and intermittent game trail that goes northeast and mostly downhill across a steep, mostly open slope for about 0.6 mile to a second, even prettier, multitiered waterfall on Boulder Creek. Several other falls on smaller creeks are nearby, but these two dramatic cascades are the highlights of this side trip.

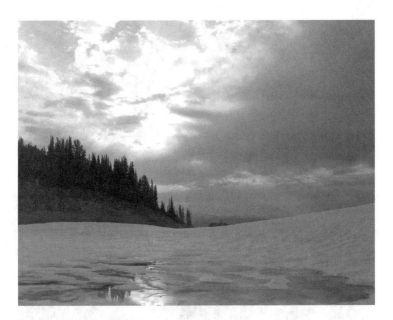

Pond south of Panhandle Gap at sunrise

Back at the saddle, you leave the ridgetop, but keep descending steeply across a wildflower-covered meadow. The trail includes several short switchbacks as it drops through the meadow and into forested terrain before bottoming out at Indian Bar. There are no views of Mount Rainier from this remarkably flat little paradise, but the surrounding cliffs support dozens of waterfalls, and the wildflowers in August are incredibly abundant. The trail crosses the meadow—with its waving grasses, gravel beds, and wildflowers—to a junction just before a bridge over the Ohanapecosh "River" (just a good-sized creek at this point). The trail to the left goes to deservedly popular Indian Bar Camp.

The main trail crosses the bridge immediately above thunderous Wauhaukaupauken Falls, a mouthful of a name that is attached to a lovely waterfall, which cannot be seen from the trail. On the other side of the bridge a short spur trail

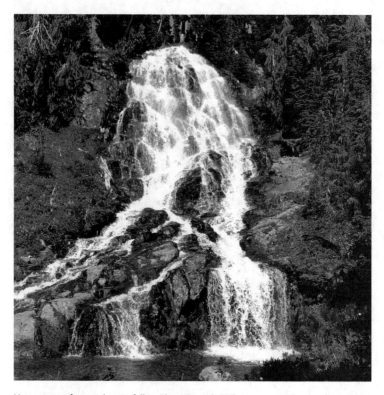

Upper part of second waterfall in Ohanapecosh Park

goes right to a large and picturesque stone shelter that is well worth a visit.

The Wonderland Trail keeps left at this junction and soon begins climbing once again. The moderately steep ascent crosses open slopes where every step reveals more of the glacier-draped mountain that has been the focus of most of your hike. After gaining about 700 feet you level out at a rolling meadow. The trail then curves to the southeast before rapidly climbing for another 0.4 mile through a mix of forest and steep meadows on a rounded ridgeline.

At 1.3 miles from Indian Bar the trail tops out on a 5,930-foot knoll and . . . well . . . *wow!* The view from this spot may be the best in the park, and it's my favorite place on the mountain to rest or eat lunch. In the distance to the south are the rugged peaks of the Goat Rocks Wilderness and the bulky volcanic cone of Mount Adams. On really clear days you can even see the sharp, snowy pinnacle of Mount Hood in Oregon, fully 100 miles away. To the southwest is the jagged ridge of the Tatoosh Range. To the east are the numerous peaks and ridges on the eastern edge of Mount Rainier National Park and in the William O. Douglas Wilderness. To the northeast are the sharp spires of the Cowlitz Chimneys. But you may not notice *any* of these things because drawing your attention like a huge, snow-covered magnet is Mount Rainier to the

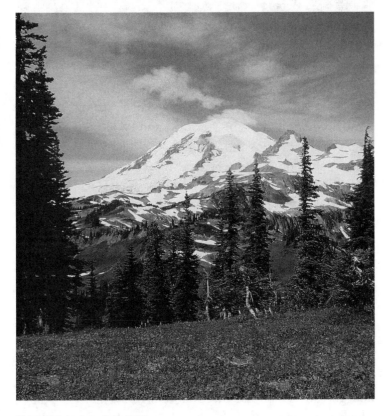

Mount Rainier from Peak 5,930

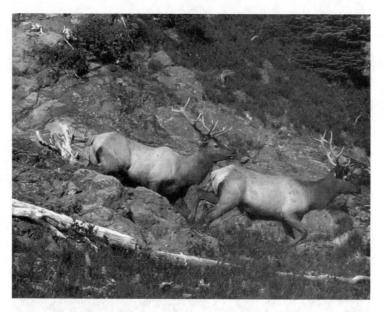

Two bull elk at Ohanapecosh Park

northwest. Little Tahoma graces the larger mountain's right flanks, while Ingraham, Cowlitz, and Whitman Glaciers, among others, tumble down the sides of the mountain in white splendor. An abundance of wildflowers—including lupine, phlox, partridgefoot, Cusick's speedwell, saxifrage, bear grass, and pink heather—add color to the scene and to the foreground of magnificent photographs. This is a place you will not soon forget.

From this high point the trail works its way south-southeast along Cowlitz Divide. The route includes lots of often steep ups and downs, and while there is actually more downhill than up, it may not seem that way to tired backpackers. Occasional switchbacks are along the way as the trail winds back and forth between the east and west sides of the ridge and goes over at least three more significant high points. Much of the distance is in open forest and meadows where you stand a good chance of seeing wildlife, including coyotes, grouse, black bears, and elk. In fact this is probably the best place along the Wonderland Trail to see elk, and you will likely at least notice their tracks and/or smell their distinctive part-musk-part-urine odor. You reach the last significant high point along the ridge at 2.1 miles from the first one, and then make a steep downhill before things level out for 0.1 mile to a junction with Cowlitz Divide Trail (the end of the Eastside Trail alternative discussed beginning on the next page).

You go straight and make a very brief climb over the top of Cowlitz Divide. From here the trail winds fairly steeply down 18 switchbacks and a few other rounded turns, always remaining faithfully in the forest on the west side of the ridge. Views are limited to a few obstructed glimpses of Mount Rainier and the Tatoosh Range. Shortly before the bottom of the descent there is a junction with the spur trail to Nickel Creek Camp, which is on the left. The Wonderland Trail continues straight for 0.1 mile to a log bridge over clear Nickel Creek. The trail then contours across wooded slopes for 0.4 mile and then steadily descends for another 0.4 mile to a junction with a dirt spur trail. The trail to the left descends for about 40 yards to the Stevens Canyon Road (also known as Washington Highway 706), which you can see and hear below you. The short detour to the parking lot at the Box Canyon Trailhead is worth the extra couple of minutes because here you'll find a restroom and a trash can. The Wonderland Trail goes straight at the junction and in just 50 yards reaches a junction with a paved nature trail coming up from the trailhead.

Section 8

Fryingpan Creek/Summerland Trailhead to Cowlitz Divide and Box Canyon via the Eastside Trail

DISTANCE..23.0 miles

Though not the scenic equivalent of the Wonderland Trail, the Eastside alternative is a very attractive route and is especially appealing early in the summer, when a significant part of the much higher Wonderland Trail is still buried under snow. It is also nice when it rains because the route is better protected by forest and less exposed to the weather than the Wonderland Trail. In addition, the waterfalls and old-growth forests that highlight this route are just as attractive under heavy cloud cover as they are in the sunshine. Finally, this somewhat longer alternative route is less popular than the Wonderland Trail, so it is easier to obtain a permit for the camps along the way.

The Eastside alternative begins with a short road walk as you go east along the White River Road from the Fryingpan Creek/Summerland Trailhead. In the summer the road has lots of traffic, so be careful because there is very little shoulder and no paralleling trail for pedestrians. After 0.6 mile you reach the Owyhigh Lakes Trailhead.

Take the Owyhigh Lakes Trail, which departs on the south side of the road across from a small parking lot. The path is wide and well maintained as it steadily ascends a forested hillside at a well-graded, moderate pace. A total of six long, lazy switchbacks keep the uphill relatively gentle. Though the forest floor is fairly open, the canopy remains dense, so while you'll enjoy plenty of shade, there are no views. At about 3 miles from the White River Road, shortly after you cross a log bridge over a small, rock-strewn creek, is the turnoff to pleasant Tamanos Creek Camp.

Beyond the Tamanos Creek Camp turnoff, the trail levels off for the next 0.6 mile, soon leaving the forest and entering lovely, wildflower-covered meadows that lead to the Owyhigh Lakes. There are two lakes, one little more than a deep pond and the other a larger but shallower lake. Both feature great views across the water to the extremely rugged spires of Governors Ridge. The trail passes above the lakes on a grassy hillside, but it is easy to wander down through meadows to the water.

Just 0.2 mile past the Owyhigh Lakes you top a partly forested pass and begin a long downhill. Though mostly in forest, the first mile or so of the descent includes some nice meadows and breaks in the trees where there are fine views to the southwest of the jagged Cowlitz Chimneys and south to tall Double Peak. The trail remains faithfully on the north side of Kotsuck Creek, though you are rarely close enough to the stream to see its clear waters or even to hear it cascading along below you.

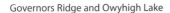

Governors Ridge and Owyhigh Lake

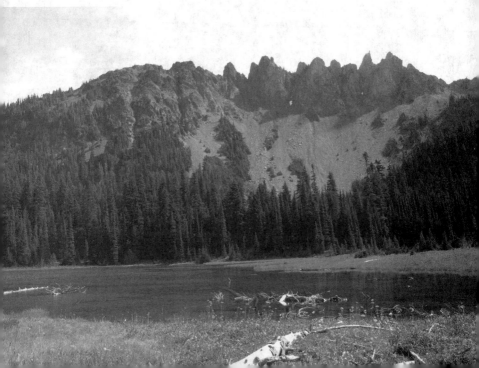

After a couple of longer switchbacks the trail makes a long, traversing descent and then a series of more than a dozen short switchbacks in increasingly dense forest. About 3.7 miles from the high point near Owyhigh Lakes, you pass near an unnamed waterfall on Kotsuck Creek, then take a log bridge over Boundary Creek, and finally enjoy a gentle descent through forests of western hemlocks and Douglas firs to a junction with the Eastside Trail. You go right, walk 0.1 mile through forest, and then take a pair of bridges over amazingly clear Chinook and Deer Creeks before reaching another junction.

You go right (south), still on the Eastside Trail, and just 75 yards later pass the signed spur trail that goes left to tiny Deer Creek Camp. The gently downhill Eastside Trail goes straight at this junction and continues south mostly in forest but at one point traveling through an open area, where you can look to the left and see Washington Highway 123 on the

Ohanapecosh Falls

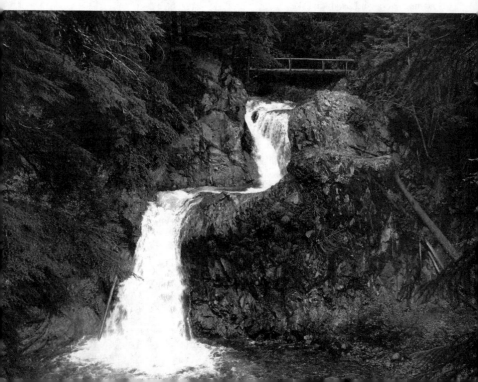

hillside above you. Although you will occasionally hear traffic from the busy thoroughfare, the sounds are not overly intrusive and do not detract significantly from your hike. About 0.8 mile from Deer Creek Camp is a bridge over Chinook Creek above a series of lovely cascades and deep pools.

The path resumes its gentle downhill course, crossing a few small side creeks along the way that add variety to the otherwise unbroken forest. Just 0.6 mile past the bridge you pass unseen, but easily heard, Stafford Falls. A boot path goes 80 yards to the left for those who want to see the short but attractive falls and the large, deep pool at its base. The forests in this area are very attractive, with a dense canopy of Douglas firs, western hemlocks, and a few western red cedars towering over lush undergrowth that is dominated by Oregon grapes, sword ferns, vanilla leaf plants, huckleberries, deer ferns, and thimbleberries. In the fall there are numerous species of colorful and interesting mushrooms.

The hiking remains unspectacular but very pleasant until a point just less than 3 miles from Deer Creek Camp, where you reach the Ohanapecosh River. Here a log bridge takes you over the stream just above Ohanapecosh Falls. The beautiful, twisting cascade is in a lovely forest setting and cries out for a rest stop and photographs. The best views are about 100 yards down the trail on the south side of the crossing.

The Eastside Trail continues south from Ohanapecosh Falls, generally heading downhill but with plenty of small ups and downs along the way. The entire distance is in forest on the hillside well above the Ohanapecosh River. For variety along the way you cross several small side creeks that are clear, splashing, and delightful. At 6.3 miles from Deer Creek Camp is a junction.

SIDE TRIP ALERT:
GROVE OF THE PATRIARCHS

The easy, short, and often crowded trail to the Grove of the Patriarchs really should not be missed as it visits the most impressive stand of old trees in the park. To take it, turn left at the junction and, 30 yards later, cross a narrow, swinging bridge over the river. Signs direct people to cross one at a time and to refrain from bouncing on the bridge when others are trying to cross. Once across the river a loop trail and partial boardwalk take you through an impressive cathedral grove of giant Douglas firs and western red cedars that are more than 1,000 years old. Interpretive signs provide interesting natural-history information about the grove and the park's forest ecosystems.

The Eastside Trail continues straight at the Grove of the Patriarchs junction and follows the crystal clear–to–emerald green Ohanapecosh River for 0.3 mile to the Grove of the Patriarchs Trailhead on the Stevens Canyon Road (also known as Washington Highway 706). The quickest way to continue with the Eastside alternative route is to turn right, following the road shoulder. After 0.5 mile of uphill you reach the signed Cowlitz Divide Trailhead.

SIDE TRIP ALERT: SILVER FALLS

A longer and more scenic way to reach this same point allows you to visit Silver Falls. To take this route, cross the highway at the Grove of the Patriarchs Trailhead and continue hiking south on the Eastside Trail. For the next 0.5 mile the path takes you through dense forest and past a series of chutes and waterfalls on the Ohanapecosh River to a junction. To reach Silver Falls, veer left and walk gradually downhill for 120 yards to where a possibly unsigned path goes left to a viewpoint beside the photogenic falls.

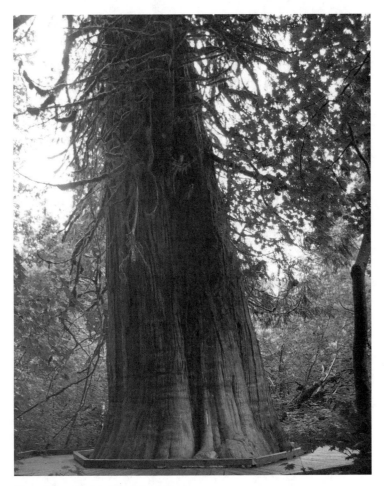

Giant cedar at Grove of the Patriarchs

After returning to the junction 120 yards from Silver Falls, turn sharply left (south) and walk a wide and gentle trail for 150 yards to a second junction. Turn right here and ascend through forest for 0.3 mile to WA 706 and the Cowlitz Divide Trailhead. Including the short side trip to Silver Falls, this alternate way of reaching this point is about 1 mile, or 0.5 mile longer than the route along the road shoulder.

From WA 706 the Cowlitz Divide Trail ascends steadily but not steeply on a forested hillside. After a little less than 1 mile the pace of your climb picks up noticeably just before the trail ascends four short switchbacks. At the top of the switchbacks a bit more moderately steep climbing in forest leads to a signed junction, 2.8 miles from WA 706. The trail to the right goes 0.1 mile to Olallie Creek Camp, a pleasantly shady spot on the north side of its namesake stream. The main trail goes straight at the junction and soon resumes climbing. A few heather plants on the forest floor and increasing numbers of mountain hemlock trees provide evidence that you are returning to a higher-elevation environment. At 1.3 miles from Olallie Creek Camp you reach the top of Cowlitz Divide and a junction with the Wonderland Trail. To complete the hike to Box Canyon, go left and follow the directions given in the previous section that describes the Wonderland Trail.

Section 9

Box Canyon to Longmire

DISTANCE...13.1 miles

The southern traverse from Box Canyon to Longmire has gotten a bad rap over the years from those who complain that it's never far from roads and not very attractive. Sure, this section suffers by comparison to other parts of the Wonderland Trail, but that is a *really* high standard. The truth is that this is a very pleasant and attractive hike with some of the trail's best

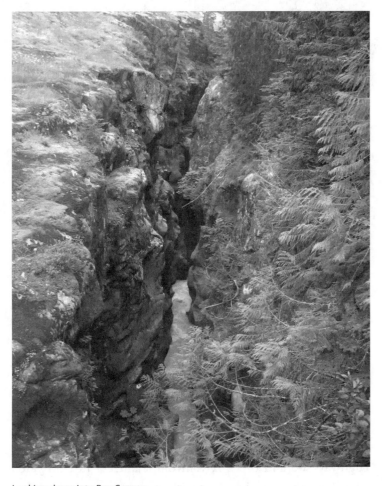

Looking down into Box Canyon

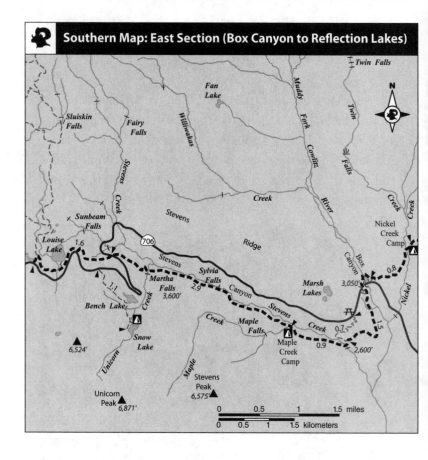

Southern Map: East Section (Box Canyon to Reflection Lakes)

waterfalls, finest forests, and prettiest lakes. Place it almost anywhere else in the country and it would draw rave reviews. It is only after being spoiled by the grandness over the previous several days that some hikers find this section to be less appealing. Appreciated for what it is, the southern traverse is a fun and quite beautiful hike that makes a good wind-down section as you head for home at Longmire.

Thru-hikers reach Box Canyon by going straight at a junction with a dirt spur trail that goes 40 yards down to Washington Highway 706 and the Box Canyon Trailhead. Just 50 yards later they come to a junction with the paved nature trail that starts at the same trailhead. Section hikers will reach this junction by walking 80 yards up the paved nature trail that starts on the east side of the bridge over Muddy Fork Cowlitz River. In either case, immediately surrounding this junction is a fascinating area of glacially polished rock, now covered with a thin surface of moss. The opening in the forest here offers nice views to the northwest of Mount Rainier.

Go straight (north) on the paved nature trail, which is bordered on either side by a wooden fence, and 0.1 mile later come to a bridge over the Muddy Fork Cowlitz River. A stop here is definitely called for to marvel at the deep and very narrow gorge of Box Canyon, which has been carved by the river into the dark volcanic rock. It is 115 feet down to the surface of the water and quite an impressive sight. The paved trail turns left (downstream) immediately after the bridge and goes about 80 yards to a possibly unsigned fork.

The paved nature trail goes straight and soon returns to WA 706. You, however, bear right (uphill) on the dirt Wonderland Trail. The path climbs two quick switchbacks and then crosses the highway where the cars go through a tunnel. About 100 yards later is a signed junction. The path to the right is a 200-foot spur trail to the highway on the west side of the tunnel.

You continue straight and go mostly downhill through dense forest, crossing a very small creek after 0.2 mile. About 1.5 miles from the Box Canyon Trailhead is a junction with Stevens Creek Trail, which goes to the right. You turn left, staying on the Wonderland Trail, and less than 100 yards later cross a bridge over Stevens Creek. The frothing stream tumbles over a cluster of huge, light-gray boulders beneath the bridge. Water action over the millennia has ground down the edges of the boulders, so they are now remarkably smooth.

Now begins an extended, mostly gentle uphill under the cover of a lovely forest. Vine maples, vanilla leaf plants, star Solomon's seal plants, various ferns, and a host of other greenery compete to find light beneath the forest canopy. After 0.9 mile you come to pleasant Maple Creek Camp.

The Wonderland Trail crosses clear Maple Creek on a log bridge immediately after the camp and proceeds up the canyon of Stevens Creek. The large stream is notorious for flooding, so you should expect to cross one or two areas of flood damage with lots of boulders and downed trees. These openings in the forest allow you to see the road high on the hillside north of the creek. Fortunately, the road is unobtrusive and does not destroy your wilderness experience. Unless trail crews have cleared it recently, thick brush (including some stinging nettles—beware) is often a problem on this section of trail. Expect to get soaked by the overhanging vegetation if things are wet from a recent rain.

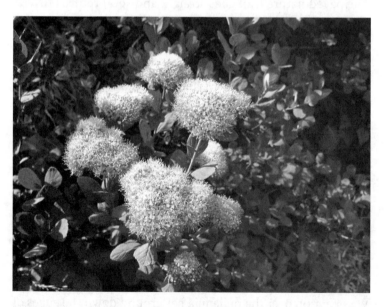

Mountain spiraea

At 1.1 miles from Maple Creek you'll hear a roar on your right signifying Sylvia Falls, a pretty, fan-shaped drop on Stevens Creek. Continuing on, you'll find that over the next mile much of the trail is on relatively exposed rocky slopes, which can be hot on sunny afternoons. There is also one spot that is particularly prone to landslides, causing regular problems for trail crews who are forced to reconstruct the tread. Ask rangers about the latest conditions on this short but potentially dangerous section.

At about 2 miles from Maple Creek is the log crossing of Unicorn Creek directly below Martha Falls. The waterfall was named after Martha Longmire, the daughter-in-law of

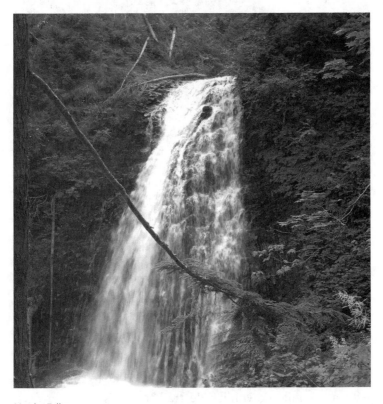

Martha Falls

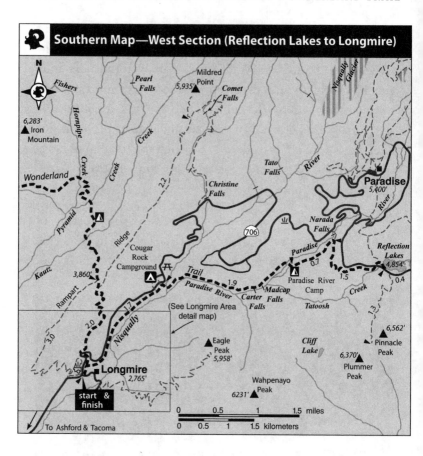

Southern Map—West Section (Reflection Lakes to Longmire)

James Longmire, an early settler and businessman on Mount Rainier. Based solely on her namesake, Ms. Longmire must have been a real beauty because this veillike falls is one of the most attractive in the park.

After a couple of quick switchbacks the trail above Martha Falls makes a steady, moderately steep uphill, mostly in forest, for 0.9 mile to a crossing of WA 706. The trail then steeply climbs a brushy hillside for just less than 0.5 mile before once again briefly touching (but not crossing) the highway. You parallel the road for 0.2 mile and then come to the junction with a 0.1-mile downhill side trail to Louise Lake, a deep jewellike lake set beneath rocky crags.

The Wonderland Trail goes straight at the Louise Lake junction. Initially the route stays in the forest below the road, but then it climbs a mostly open huckleberry-covered hillside where you can look down on sparkling Louise Lake. At the top of this climb is a junction with the eastern end of the Lakes Trail. You go straight and not quite 0.2 mile later reach WA 706 beside the easternmost of the Reflection Lakes. These lakes are a favorite photo spot for park visitors, and the scene is no less photogenic for being shared with car-bound tourists. The route takes you past the Reflection Lakes with their famous views of Mount Rainier as you follow the highway shoulder going west for the next 0.4 mile. Along the way the Pinnacle Peak Trail takes off to the south, but you stick with the road shoulder until the trail resumes at the end of a stone wall that lines the parking area for Reflection Lakes. There may be no sign here, but the trail is obvious going downhill to the right on the north side of the road.

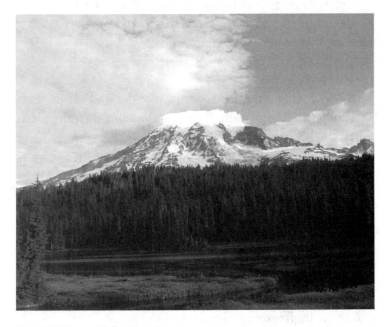

Mount Rainier over Reflection Lake

The path follows the somewhat marshy shore of the largest (westernmost) Reflection Lake for less than 0.2 mile, crosses the outlet creek on a bridge, and then comes to a junction with the western end of the Lakes Trail. You go left and 0.1 mile later cross WA 706 to its south side.

From here the trail closely parallels the road, staying in the meadows and forest directly below the highway for about 0.6 mile. You then round the top of a minor ridge and descend four moderately graded switchbacks to a junction with Narada Falls Trail.

> **SIDE TRIP ALERT:** NARADA FALLS
>
> Even though you'll have to share it with lots of car tourists, do not miss the short side trip to the viewpoint of Narada Falls. This 168-foot, veillike drop on the Paradise River is extremely beautiful and quite photogenic. The trail goes to the right at the junction and reaches the viewpoint in less than 0.1 mile, so it should take only a few well-rewarded minutes.

The now wide and brush-free Wonderland Trail goes sharply left at the Narada Falls junction and then descends fairly steeply through attractive but viewless forest. After 0.7 mile you come to the turnoff for Paradise River Camp, which is a pleasant and shady spot to spend the night. About 90 yards after the camp turnoff, a bridge crosses the crystal-clear waters of Paradise River. A relatively gentle descent for the next 0.7 mile takes you to sliding and very pretty Madcap Falls, and then less than 0.1 mile later to thundering Carter Falls. It's a little difficult to get a full view of the crashing falls through the intervening trees, but what you can see is impressive.

From Carter Falls the trail descends in a stair-step fashion for the next 1.1 miles, alternating fairly steep sections with parts that are quite gentle. An interesting feature starting about 0.2 mile below Carter Falls is a large, wooden pipe, immediately on the right side of the trail. Many decades ago the pipe supplied the water to turn a hydroelectric generator at the long-abandoned Eagle Rock Mine.

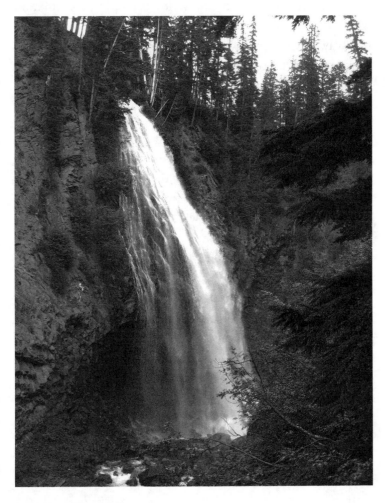

Looking up at Narada Falls

At the bottom of the descent is the Nisqually River, a rushing and heavily silt-laden stream that you cross on a long log bridge. As with so many streams along the Wonderland Trail the exact location of the bridge changes from year to year as the river's channel moves around with each spring flood.

On the other side of the river you make a very brief climb to the Carter Falls Trailhead on WA 706. The Wonderland Trail veers left away from the trailhead parking lot and heads southwest through forest for 0.1 mile to a junction with the first of two spur trails that go right and cross the highway to Cougar Rock Campground. Unlike White River Campground, there are no designated backpacker campsites at this car campground. If you plan to stay here, you'll have to compete for a spot with car campers and pay the same fee as they do for a site.

The main trail goes straight at the junction and continues very gradually, descending under the shady canopy of large western hemlocks and Douglas firs. As will be true the rest of the way to Longmire, you will frequently hear, and sometimes see, cars zipping by on WA 706 on your right. A more constant (and more pleasantly natural) sound is the rushing Nisqually River, not far to your left. You pass the second spur trail to Cougar Rock Campground about 0.15 mile after the first, after which the trail remains in the sometimes very narrow strip of forest between the river and the road all the way to the junction at the start of the grand loop. Turn left and in 0.1 mile return to Longmire and the end of your long, glorious hike of a lifetime.

Appendix A:
Recommended Reading

Given its prominence and beloved status in the Pacific Northwest, it's not surprising that Mount Rainier has inspired countless books covering almost every conceivable aspect of the mountain's human history, plants and animals, weather, hiking trails, wildflowers, geology, volcanic origins, climbing routes, and pretty much anything else you could imagine. The following are some of the more interesting, useful, or entertaining tomes that are worthy of your time and attention.

Hiking and Climbing Guides

Gauthier, Mike. *Mount Rainier: A Climbing Guide, Second Edition.* Seattle: Mountaineers Books, 2005.

Nelson, Dan. *Day Hiking Mount Rainier: National Park Trails.* Seattle: Mountaineers Books, 2008.

Natural History Books

Blackwell, Laird R. *Wildflowers of Mount Rainier.* Auburn, WA: Lone Pine Publishing, 2000.

Dreimiller, Joe. *A Pocket Field Guide to the Plants and Animals of Mount Rainier.* Seattle: Elton-Wolf Publishing, 1999.

Pringle, Patrick T. *Roadside Geology of Mount Rainier National Park and Vicinity.* Olympia, WA: Washington Division of Geology and Earth Resources, 2008.

History, Literature, and Others

Barcott, Bruce. *The Measure of a Mountain: Beauty and Terror on Mount Rainier.* Seattle: Sasquatch Books, 1997.

Filley, Bette. *The Big Fact Book about Mount Rainier: Fascinating Facts, Records, Lists, Topics, Characters and Stories.* Issaquah, WA: Dunamis House, 1996.

Schmoe, Floyd. *A Year in Paradise.* Seattle: Mountaineers Books, 1999.

Smith, Allan H. *Takhoma: Ethnography of Mount Rainier National Park.* Pullman, WA: Washington State University Press, 2006.

Appendix B:
Selected Area Restaurants,
Motels, Outdoors Stores,
and Other Businesses

As mentioned earlier, if you need to purchase last-minute food, cooking fuel, or other hiking supplies, it is much better (and cheaper) to buy them before you get into or near Mount Rainier National Park, where the selection of such supplies is limited. In the Seattle-Tacoma area there are dozens of excellent outdoors retailers. Two REI stores are particularly convenient for those who are flying into Seattle to do the Wonderland Trail:

REI Southcenter/Tukwila
240 Andover Park W
Tukwila, WA 98188
(206) 248-1938
rei.com

(in the Southcenter Shopping Center just east of I-5 where Washington Highway 518 comes in from the west out of Seattle-Tacoma International Airport)

REI Tacoma
3825 South Steele Street
Tacoma, WA 98409
(253) 671-1938
(off Exit 131 just east of I-5)

Hikers traveling from the Seattle area to Longmire will pass through the tourist-oriented town of Ashford just a few miles before coming to the park's southwest entrance. This small community has a variety of motels, gift shops, and similar businesses that cater to people heading for the mountain. A complete listing of motels and other businesses is available online from various Yellow Pages services. A few of the more popular and interesting locations include:

Alexander's Country Inn & Restaurant

37515 Washington Highway 706 E
Ashford, WA 98304
(360) 569-2300

alexanderscountryinn.com

The lodging is in a historic Victorian manor with individually designed rooms. The place is rather expensive but very quaint. The inn also has a day spa. The restaurant has *outstanding* homemade desserts and is well worth a stop just for these tasty sweets!

Mountain Meadows Inn Bed & Breakfast

28912 Washington Highway 706
Ashford, WA 98304
(360) 569-2788

mountainmeadowsinn.com

This B&B is in a wonderful forested setting with many nature trails around the property.

Highlander Steak House

30319 Washington Highway 706 E
Ashford, WA 98304
(360) 569-2953

They serve better-than-average steaks, but the clientele can be a bit seedy, especially on weekends.

Wild Berry Restaurant

37718 Washington Highway 706 E

Ashford, WA 98304

(360) 569-2277

This small restaurant is especially well known for its baked goods and desserts.

Ex-Nihilo (Recycled Spirits of Iron Sculpture Park)

22410 Washington Highway 706

Ashford, WA 98304

(360) 569-8804

danielklennert.com

For a change of pace that is surprisingly worth your time, an interesting stop just a couple of miles west of Ashford is Ex-Nihilo, also known as the Recycled Spirits of Iron Sculpture Park. Here local artist Dan Klennert displays a wide selection of his fascinating sculptures made with recycled wheels, parts from broken-down appliances, pieces of old farm equipment, and other stray bits of metal. Admission is free, and you can often see the artist at work.

Appendix C:
Park Service Website and
Telephone Numbers

The website for Mount Rainier National Park is **nps.gov/ mora.** Once you are on this website you can navigate to all kinds of useful information about the latest trail conditions, road and trail closures, obtaining a permit reservation form, fees, and so on.

For hikers, the most useful telephone numbers in the park are:

Carbon River Ranger Station: (360) 829-9639

Longmire Museum: (360) 569-6575

Longmire Wilderness Information Center: (360) 569-6650

Paradise Guide House (for climbing information): (360) 569-6641

White River Wilderness Information Center: (360) 569-6670

Index

About the Author

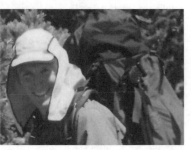

photographed by Becky Lovejoy

Douglas Lorain's family moved to the Pacific Northwest in 1969, and he has been obsessively hitting the trails of his home region ever since. Over the years he calculates that he has logged well more than 30,000 trail miles in this corner of the continent, including several hundred doing (and redoing) the spectacular trails of Mount Rainier National Park. Despite a history that includes being shot at by a hunter, bitten by a rattlesnake, charged by grizzly bears (twice!)—don't worry, none of these happened on Mount Rainier—and donating countless gallons of blood to "invertebrate vampires" (OK, at least a few pints of those happened on Mount Rainier), he happily sees no end in sight.

Lorain is a photographer and recipient of the National Outdoor Book Award. His books cover only the best from the thousands of hikes and backpacking trips he has taken throughout Idaho, Oregon, Washington, Wyoming, and elsewhere. When pressed, however, he admits that it would be hard to find anything in all those miles that is better than the Wonderland Trail. His other guidebook titles include *100 Classic Hikes in Oregon, Backpacking Idaho, Backpacking Oregon, Backpacking Washington, Backpacking Wyoming, One Night Wilderness: Portland,* and *Afoot & Afield Portland/Vancouver.*

Although he considers his real home to be on the trail, those days he is forced to stay indoors, he lives in Portland, Oregon, with his wife, Becky Lovejoy.